THE 8TH DAY:

My Journey through Kidney Failure

Marc A. Pouhé

Prologue:
THE 8TH DAY
Chapter 1: The Journey Begins
Chapter 2: The Emergency Room
Chapter 3: A New Reality
Chapter 4: The Procedure
Chapter 5: Visitors and Progress
Chapter 6: Small Victories
Chapter 7: The Road Ahead
Chapter 8: Progress and Preparations
Chapter 9: New Beginnings and Harsh Realities
Chapter 10: Family, Progress, and New Horizons
Chapter 11: Hurdles and Hope (Part 1 Revised)
Chapter 11: Hurdles and Hope (Part 1)
Chapter 11: Hurdles and Hope (Part 2 Revised)
Chapter 12: Under the Microscope
Chapter 13: A Journey Within
Chapter 14: The Waiting Game
Chapter 15: A Beacon of Hope
Chapter 16: The Heart of the Matter
Chapter 17: After the Procedure: A Moment of Relief
Chapter 18: Wheels of Freedom: Leaving the Hospital
Chapter 19: Bridging Distances: A Father-Daughter Moment
Chapter 20: The Verdict: A Step Closer to New Life
Chapter 21: Listening to the Body
Chapter 22: The Waiting Game
Chapter 23: The Gift and The Wait
Chapter 24: The Call and The Promise: A New Chapter Begins
Chapter 25: The Long Wait: June's Bitter Truth
Chapter 26: Summer of Uncertainty
Chapter 27: The Call That Changed Everything
A Perspective on Waiting

Prologue:

At first glance, my current story of kidney failure and transplantation seems relatively recent. In actuality, my journey began in May 2009, when I was diagnosed with IgA Nephropathy, or Immunoglobulin A Nephropathy. I'll do my best not to overload you with undefined medical jargon. To be honest, in 2009, it took me well over a month to properly pronounce "nephropathy" or "nephrologist." In short, IgA Nephropathy is a kidney disease characterized by an overly aggressive immune system, often caused by undiagnosed or untreated strep throat.

The body produces tough Immunoglobulin A molecules that go to work, annihilating the strep and protecting you. The problem is, they don't stop there. Imagine your kidneys as a pasta strainer. They filter out toxins in the form of urine and send the cleaner blood back into circulation. That's one of many jobs the kidneys perform. They're also responsible for producing red blood cells, among other things. But when the large, aggressive IgA molecules reach the pasta strainer, they're like hot nickels punching holes in the neat, existing openings. Large, irreparable holes. So if you imagine a pasta strainer (healthy kidney) normally holding back pasta (clean blood) and dumping out dirty water (toxins and urine), those hot nickel holes (IgA molecules) would essentially render the pasta strainer permanently useless.

That's what made me sick in 2009. That's why I was on hemodialysis from 2010 to 2012, and that's why I received my first kidney transplant in 2012. The summer after my transplant, I became a writer for a local arts magazine. One assignment was to write a short article about myself and my experience. Finding an old piece of your own writing is like stepping into a time machine, but I believe sharing this draft is the best way to fill you in on years of background.

"Marc Pouhé is enjoying the renewed energy and vigor that comes with a kidney transplant. He is the recipient of a new kidney thanks to his youngest brother Jacques Pouhe and a six person, three way kidney exchange that took place on June 1, 2012 at the Texas Transplant Institute in San Antonio, Texas.

Marc was diagnosed with end stage renal disease in May of 2009 due to IgA Nephropathy, a kidney disease in which the body's own immune system attacks the kidneys causing permanent damage in Marc's case. Before his diagnosis, Marc was an award winning stage and film actor based out of Austin, Texas.

Marc discovered acting at Tulane University when a friend suggested he audition for William Shakespeare's Pericles. He quickly became a student of classical theatre and contemporary drama but also excelled in musical roles such as Chicago's Billy Flynn.

Marc launched his professional acting career in 2004 and has worked extensively with Austin's finest theatre organizations including Zach Theatre, Austin Shakespeare, Pro Arts Collective, and Mary Moody Northen Theatre at St. Edward's University.

Theatre credits include title characters in Macbeth and Othello, leading roles in Chicago, Six Degrees of Separation, Death and the King's Horseman, Master Harold...and the Boys, and supporting roles in Urinetown, Jesus Christ Superstar, Take Me Out, The Exonerated, The Grapes of Wrath, Three Sisters, Cyrano de Bergerac, The Glass Menagerie, and several others. Marc is a three-time winner of the Austin Critics' Table Award and is a three-time nominee for the B. Iden Payne Acting Award.

In 2006, Marc expanded his focus to include film and television. He's appeared on Fox's Prison Break and NBC's Friday Night Lights. Film credits include The Overbrook Brothers, Between Kings and Queens, Mnemosyne Rising, Play Time, The Ticket, Holy Hell, and Jesse's Closet. Marc is also the voice of Dogbert on the animated web series on Dilbert.com.

Marc underwent a major life change after being diagnosed with chronic kidney failure, following an award winning performance as wayward preacher James Casey in The Grapes of Wrath at Zach Theatre in May 2009. He moved to Harlingen shortly after being diagnosed so that his mother, a pharmacist, could help guide and manage his treatment.

Marc was introduced to his nephrologist, Dr. Oladayo Sanusi, in January of 2010. It is this doctor/patient relationship that influenced and encouraged Marc to begin painting again. He finds the creative outlet provided by painting to be an excellent surrogate for the creative rewards provided by acting.

One of Marc's earliest pieces is entitled Sicklist and is a visual representation of his journey with IgA nephropathy and several of the secondary symptoms and diseases that accompanied his kidney failure.

The three years that Marc dealt with end stage renal disease were physically and emotionally challenging to say the least. The most difficult times were the first two years, with the rapid progression of his illness from May 2009 until starting dialysis in June 2010, and then the frequent trips to the hospital from June 2010 until December of 2011.

But in mid December of 2011, things took a change for the better. Marc's youngest brother Jacques was in from New York completing final cross matching for the donation. Even though Marc and Jacques were not a blood match, the Texas Transplant Institute decided to include them in a revolutionary kidney swap program. This was welcome news as Marc had spent the previous year waiting on a matched live donor that was eventually disqualified.

The possibility of a swap was initially scheduled for January 2012. This change in status inspired Marc to begin painting his first new work in six years, a Christmas present for his mother, a 24 by 48 inch family portrait. He also painted a portrait for his brother. With renewed confidence and inspiration, Marc began a creative journey over the next six months that produced over 90 new works of art.

The pieces included abstract paintings, circular and rectangular pieces influenced by Kandinsky and Mondrian, Haitian scenes influenced by his mother's heritage, mathematical themes, and photo realistic recreations of churches and architecture. Marc was driven by the possibility of improving health, and even when the initial swap fell through in January, he continued painting, improving daily and teaching himself new techniques.

The final swap materialized on June 1, 2012. Six total patients, three donors and three recipients participated in a successful morning surgery. The day before the transplant Marc was interviewed by Judyth Piazza for the radio program American Perspectives about his journey through kidney failure and his new found success as a visual artist.

The weeks since Marc's transplant have been some of the most creative and production times in his life. While in the hospital in mid June for a week-long follow up for a post transplant complication, Marc decided to create new art on the dry erase board in his hospital room, creating new fans of the medical and nursing staff at the Texas Transplant Institute.

Upon returning home at the end of June, Marc produced five short films detailing and chronicling his experiences with kidney failure, visual arts, his professional acting career, and a look back at his childhood. These films combine to form a 30 minute short available for viewing on Marc's YouTube channel marcpouhe.

Marc is also preparing for his first art gallery showing on August 11, 2012 for RGVArtOnline in Harlingen, Texas at the Golden Palms Resort.

Physically, Marc is recovering nicely, thanks to the outstanding care of his primary nephrologist Dr. Oladayo Sanusi, and the Texas Transplant Institute Team including Drs. Kaputzchek, Bingamman, and Wright. The nursing staff at TTI and the dialysis staff at DaVita Valley Baptist in Harlingen, Texas all deserve a big round of applause as well. A twice daily round of exercise is also playing a big part in Marc's successful recovery.

Marc has also started writing a novel, untitled as of yet but a brief sample follows:

The weekend came and went. Monday came and went. Michael had put off the doctor's office because since the play ended he wasn't receiving weekly paychecks. His salary had to be invoiced, routed through his agent, and in his pocket any time from 2 to 8 weeks after each job was completed. So cash on hand was low. It was Tuesday and the weight gain was close to 50 lbs now. All water. It was hard for him to breathe and between Karen and the pharmacist's suggestions, Michael was about to scrounge up whatever cash he had and go to the doctor. He would go first thing Wednesday morning. But he couldn't get to sleep Tuesday night.

"Karen...Karen."

"Yes, baby?"

"I can't...I can't sleep. I'm afraid. I'm scared if I fall asleep I'll stop breathing and not wake up."

"This is ridiculous. You're going to see a doctor."

"I know, I know, I put it off, but I see how important it is now. I'm just afraid I won't make it until tomorrow morning."

"Are you serious?"

"....yes."

"Listen, I'm driving you to the emergency room right now. I used to work in a hospital. They can't turn you away in the emergency room if you're really sick and trust me honey, you are sick."

"Okay."

Though Michael was 9 years older than Karen, he surrendered to her authority and listened to her instructions as if he were a scared 3rd grader.

They entered the emergency room of St. David's South Austin at about 11pm May 19, 2009. He'd only been in the hospital recently for the birth of his two children, Marc in 2004 and Angelica in 2006. And though heavily invested in both visits, he was never physically ill or at risk before. He and Karen were anticipating a long wait in triage. But Michael told the check in nurse the previously unknown magic words.

"I can't breath so well and I'm having chest pains. I gained about 50 lbs of water in the last two weeks and I'm afraid to go to sleep because I don't think I'll wake up."

If you missed it, the magic words were chest pains. Something about chest pains mobilizes medical professionals immediately. More than broken bones, more than fever, more than stab wounds. I guess because those other problems will either still be there in an hour (broken bones, stab wounds) or gone in an hour (fever, especially in infants). But chest pains can kill you if not addressed immediately.

Regardless, Michael was thankful for the unknown importance of my symptoms, in that it got him seen quickly. He began filling out and answering medical history questionnaires. They were confusing and difficult but would become second nature over the next few years.

The first nurse came in and took Michael's blood pressure: 166/95 heart rate 95. Temperature normal, 98.7. Then came a battery of tests: blood sample, urine sample, chest x-ray, ekg. Then a gentleman came in with admissions paperwork and asked Michael if he had insurance.

"No."

The administrator took a beat and asked Michael to fill out more paperwork, and took copies of his driver's license and social security card.

Michael and Karen waited for what seemed like an hour before anyone else returned. It was now 1 am. Michael was exhausted but couldn't even think of sleeping. The on-call doctor entered and introduced himself.

"Hello, Michael ... Prince is it?"

"Yes sir."

"I'm Dr. Wilson. Preliminary lab results are in and we'd like to admit you to the hospital."

"What's wrong with me?"

"Well a few things. First we found high amounts of protein and blood in your urine. Still waiting on some blood work, your ekg appears normal. But I can say with what we have so far that you have nephrotic syndrome."

"Nephrotic ..?"

"What that means is that your kidneys have reduced capacity and are pouring out protein. Your albumin count is extremely low, that's what's causing the edema or swelling in your legs."

"How do I get my albumin back?"

"Well that's the problem, it usually doesn't come back if your kidneys are damaged. We want to keep you here at least for a few days and run many more tests to see what's causing the nephrotic syndrome. We're just waiting for a bed to open upstairs and we'll get you checked in."

Though the doctor talked for at least another minute, Michael's concentration drifted off and his mind began to race. From this moment on his life would never be the same.

Marc's future is wide open with his improved health, but he intends to continue growing in the visual arts. A return to acting is a possibility down the road, an interest in taking the MCAT and pursuing a medical degree is in progress. Marc enjoys the concrete nature and permanence of his artwork and looks forward to continued growth and development in the visual arts."

Well, I never finished that novel. Which is probably for the best. But hopefully this one serves as a vehicle for a bigger message about healthcare reform, resilience, family, friendship, despair, and hope.

My current kidney failure story is that my 2012 kidney has run its course. Twelve years is not a bad run for a transplant. But I'm sick enough to require daily dialysis and I continue to wait (as of this writing) for a kidney transplant.

Also a note about this novel's creation: I actually didn't set out to write a novel.

When I became deathly ill in November 2023, as my wife Teri drove me to the hospital, I decided to start filming myself and explaining what was happening. I have three teenage and adult kids who don't live with me, and I wish I could have been in their lives more, especially when they were very young, but I moved a long distance to get the medical help I needed. This book isn't the place to litigate fault, but I personally regret not being more involved in their lives.

I was filming everything because I honestly thought I was going to die in the hospital. I wanted to create a record for my kids. And then the doctors came. And then I got a little bit better. And then friends came, unprompted. And then my mother came from hundreds of miles away. I filmed many of those interactions, even from the time I could barely speak or see clearly. I left the hospital eight days later. I kept filming.

By February 2024, my cheap, pay-as-you-go phone ran out of storage. I invested in the Samsung equivalent of the newest top-of-the-line Apple phone. I was spoiled! I was making an accidental documentary! I already had well over three hours of footage. I used a combination of apps available on my phone to edit the film down to 2 hours and whittled even more off to 1 hour 45 minutes.

Here's where the novel began. One thing that helped me see what I could cut from the film was attempting to write a screenplay in reverse. By that I mean, watching the edited footage, taking notes, pausing, writing some more, teaching myself how to format a screenplay, what to note in the scene descriptions, and trying my best to match the script with the action already captured. When I read some of the long passages from myself or friends who came and told wonderful 15-minute stories, I realized, those are great to witness in person, slightly less interesting to watch on screen, even less interesting to read in a book, and terrifying to see if you are an actor preparing to play a scene. I'm talking five to six-page stretches of monologue.

I also thought, I'd like to be able to share these messages with more people. So the best way for me to do that was to take the screenplay, keep the first-person narrative, highlight the important scenes, and combine or even drop the scenes that were no less important but would be impossible to convince an actor to do if this somehow spawns a miniseries or something in 10 years.

All of the above being said, this novel is based on a true story. It's my story, and as I'm writing this prologue it's not yet over. Not philosophically speaking, but there are literally some medical procedures that have to happen before I can write the final chapter, and I don't want to spoil the rest of the book for you this early.

Some guidelines:

- Most of the names have been changed. I believe one Dr. has the same last name but most characters have had their names changed or not used at all. Only my wife, Teri, and I have our full names.

- Some of the timing of events is shifted or combined.

- Some events are omitted and some are slightly altered for flow, not entertainment purposes.

- This is my first attempt at a multi-pronged project of this magnitude so I really hope you like it. If you don't, feel free to leave that off of the Amazon review page. But you can personally email me at marcpouhe@gmail.com to tell me to quit writing, or directing, but I'll never stop acting.

That's it! I don't know if prologues are supposed to be eleven pages long, it's my first one. I hope I gave you enough background to more fully enjoy this story. Thank you for reading this far.

Marc A. Pouhé

THE 8TH DAY

The soft strains of classical music wash over me as I contemplate the gravity of my situation. The melody feels both comforting and ominous, like a bittersweet lullaby for what might be my final days. Each note seems to resonate with the uncertainty of my future, a haunting reminder of the fragility of life. As the music fades, I'm left with the stark reality of my condition, laid bare in cold, clinical terms:

On November 8, 2023, I was admitted to St. David's Round Rock Hospital. My kidneys, those small but vital organs, had essentially given up on one of their most crucial tasks – producing red blood cells. It's a strange feeling, knowing your body is failing you in such a fundamental way. The realization hits me in waves, each one threatening to drown me in fear and despair.

In the weeks leading up to my hospitalization, I had become intimately familiar with the inside of medical facilities. Multiple blood transfusions had become a routine part of my life, each one a temporary stopgap measure against my body's inability to sustain itself. I remember the first time I needed a transfusion, the shock of seeing my own blood, so depleted, being replaced by the vibrant red of donor blood. It was a surreal experience, watching life literally being pumped back into my veins.

But even more alarming was the sudden weight gain – thirty pounds of toxic fluid building up inside me, turning my body into its own poison container. I could feel the heaviness with every move, my clothes growing tighter, my breath becoming more labored. It was as if my body was slowly drowning from the inside out.

I remember the look on my physician's face when he strongly advised me to seek immediate medical attention. The urgency in his voice, the concern in his eyes – it was then that the true gravity of my situation began to sink in. This wasn't just another complication; this was life or death. The weight of his words settled on me like a physical presence, adding to the burden my body was already struggling to bear.

As I prepare to recount the events that followed, I'm struck by the surreal nature of it all. This is my story – a chronicle of my fight for survival, my journey to secure a life-saving kidney transplant. It's a tale of fear and hope, of pain and perseverance. And as I begin to tell it, I can't help but wonder: will this be my legacy, or just another chapter in a longer story? The uncertainty of it all is both terrifying and oddly liberating. In this moment, poised on the edge of the unknown, I feel a strange mix of vulnerability and strength. Whatever comes next, I know I have no choice but to face it head-on.

Chapter 1: The Journey Begins

The car's interior feels unusually cramped today, November 8, 2023. I'm wedged into the passenger seat, my bloated body an uncomfortable reminder of my condition. The seatbelt stretches tight across my swollen abdomen, a constant pressure that serves as a physical manifestation of the weight of my illness. Next to me, my wife Teri takes the driver's seat, her face a mask of concern barely hiding her own discomfort.

I lift my cellphone, my hands shaking slightly as I position it to capture both of us in the frame. The weight of the device feels immense, or maybe it's just my weakened state making everything seem more difficult. As I start recording, I'm acutely aware that this might be the last message I leave for my three teenage children. The thought sends a chill through me, despite the unseasonably warm 80-degree weather outside. I try to push away the morbid thoughts, focusing instead on the task at hand.

"This is Teri," I say, my voice sounding foreign to my own ears, distorted and breathless. Each word is an effort, pushing past the fluid buildup that constricts my chest. "She just got diagnosed with pneumonia, is it? She's kind enough to drive me to the emergency room."

Teri gives a small, tight smile to the camera before turning her attention to the road. I can see the strain in her eyes, the worry lines etched deeply around her mouth. She's battling her own illness, yet here she is, taking care of me. The guilt mingles with gratitude, creating a complex emotional cocktail that threatens to overwhelm me.

The car pulls out of our driveway, the familiar surroundings blurring as we head towards an uncertain future. I watch our house disappear in the side mirror, wondering if I'll ever see it again. The streets we've driven countless times now seem alien, as if we're embarking on a journey to a foreign land rather than a trip to the local hospital.

The GPS voice, calm and detached, guides us to the local emergency room parking lot. Its monotonous directions feel absurdly normal in the face of our dire situation. I find myself latching onto the familiar sound, using it as an anchor to reality as my mind threatens to spiral into panic.

I turn the camera back to myself, fighting to keep my swollen eyes open. The face that looks back at me from the phone screen is barely recognizable – puffy, pale, with a sickly sheen that speaks volumes about my condition. "My doctor told us we'd be able to get an emergency port in my stomach to start dialysis," I explain, each word an effort. "I've been throwing up nonstop and lost a lot of blood internally."

As I speak, I notice the world around me seems to be losing its vibrancy. Colors fade, shadows deepen, until everything takes on a monochromatic quality. It's as if my deteriorating condition is bleeding the color from my perception of the world. This gradual desaturation feels symbolic, a visual representation of how my illness is draining the life from me, bit by bit.

The car comes to a stop in the parking lot. Teri and I exchange a look, volumes spoken in that silent moment. Despite everything, we manage to take a picture together. A memento, I think, of what I fear might be our last moments together. The click of the camera shutter sounds final, like the closing of a chapter.

As we prepare to leave the relative safety of our car for the unknown that awaits us in the emergency room, I'm struck by a wave of emotions – fear, certainly, but also a strange sense of relief. Whatever happens next, at least the waiting is over. The next steps of my journey are about to unfold, for better or worse.

I take a deep breath, wincing at the discomfort it causes, and reach for the door handle. It's time to face whatever comes next. As I step out of the car, leaning heavily on Teri for support, I silently pray that this is not the end of my story, but the beginning of a new chapter – one that leads to healing and recovery.

Chapter 2: The Emergency Room

The emergency room hits me like a sensory overload, a cacophony of sights and sounds all blurring together in my deteriorating state. The automatic doors slide open with a whoosh, releasing a blast of cold, antiseptic-scented air that makes me shiver despite the warmth of the day outside. It's as if I'm crossing a threshold into another world – one governed by the relentless rhythm of life and death.

Monitors beep incessantly, their rhythm a discordant melody of urgency. Each high-pitched tone feels like it's drilling directly into my skull, adding to the pounding headache that's been my constant companion for days. Medical staff bustle around, their movements quick and purposeful. Their scrubs, normally a rainbow of calming colors, now appear in shades of grey in my desaturated vision.

I catch glimpses of other patients, their worried faces mirroring what I imagine is my own expression. A child cries somewhere in the distance, the sound piercing through the general din. An elderly man in a wheelchair stares vacantly at the wall, his stillness a stark contrast to the frenetic energy around him. I wonder about their stories, what brought them here on this day that feels so monumental in my own life.

The check-in process is a blur of questions and paperwork. I struggle to focus, to provide the necessary information. Teri steps in, her voice steady as she explains my condition to the triage nurse. I'm grateful for her strength, even as I feel a pang of guilt for relying on her so heavily.

Someone – a nurse, I think – guides me to a bed in the back portion of the ER. The journey feels like a marathon, each step an immense effort. By the time I'm settled on the bed, I'm breathing heavily, sweat beading on my forehead despite the chill in the air.

I'm hooked up to various machines, their hums and beeps creating a symphony of modern medicine. Wires snake across my body, connecting me to monitors that will track my vital signs. A blood pressure cuff inflates periodically, its squeeze a reminder of the precariousness of my condition.

As I lie there, I can't help but fixate on my bag of medication nearby. Those little pills and vials, my lifeline for so long, seem woefully inadequate in the face of my current crisis. I think about how I used to take my health for granted, how a handful of pills seemed like such an inconvenience. Now, I'd give anything to go back to those simpler times.

Time becomes fluid, stretching and compressing unpredictably. I drift in and out of consciousness, each moment of clarity bringing a new realization of how dire my situation has become. The black and white world around me feels appropriate – my life has been reduced to this stark, binary state: survival or...the alternative.

In my more lucid moments, I observe the ER staff at work. Their efficiency is both comforting and terrifying – comforting because I know I'm in capable hands, terrifying because their urgency underscores the severity of my condition. I catch snatches of their conversations, medical jargon that I've become all too familiar with over the years of my illness.

Teri remains a constant presence at my side, her hand holding mine, grounding me in reality when the pain and fear threaten to sweep me away. I see the toll this is taking on her, the worry etched in the lines of her face, but she never wavers. Her strength becomes my strength, her hope a lifeline I cling to.

As the day wears on, a thought keeps circling in my mind: This is just the first day. How many more will there be? Will I see this through to the other side? The uncertainty is almost as debilitating as the physical symptoms. I try to focus on the present, on each breath, each moment I'm still here, still fighting.

Eventually, a doctor approaches my bed. His face is serious as he explains that I'll be admitted for further treatment. The news is both a relief and a new source of anxiety. Relief that I'll be getting the intensive care I need, anxiety about what that care will entail.

As they prepare to move me to a room, I take one last look around the ER. This place, with its constant rhythm of crisis and resolution, has been the first stage of what I now realize will be a long and difficult journey. But as they wheel me out, I feel a glimmer of hope. I've made it through this first hurdle. Whatever comes next, I'll face it with the same determination.

The ER doors close behind me, and I brace myself for the next chapter of my story.

Chapter 3: A New Reality

The next morning finds me in a hospital room, a slight improvement from the chaotic ER but no less clinical. Sunlight filters weakly through the venetian blinds, casting striped shadows across the room. The walls are a pale, institutional green that seems designed to be as inoffensive as possible. It's a color that doesn't commit to anything, much like my current state of being – suspended between illness and recovery.

I'm perched in a chair, wrapped in a hoodie despite the controlled temperature of the room. The comfort of the familiar garment is a small solace in this sterile environment. It smells faintly of home, a scent that both comforts and saddens me as I wonder when I'll return there.

The events of yesterday play on repeat in my mind – the frantic drive to the hospital, the chaos of the ER, the battery of tests and questions. It all seems like a bad dream, but the IV in my arm and the persistent beep of the heart monitor serve as constant reminders of my new reality.

I've positioned my phone to record again, determined to document this journey, whether it leads to recovery or...somewhere else. The act of recording helps me feel less powerless, gives me a sense of purpose in a situation where I have little control. It's also a way to communicate with my children, to leave them something of myself if... I push the thought away. I can't go down that road right now.

Taking a deep breath, I begin my update. "So, slight change of plans," I say, my voice stronger than yesterday but still carrying the weight of my condition. The words feel inadequate to describe the seismic shift in my treatment plan, but I press on.

"My condition has deteriorated so rapidly that we're going to switch from peritoneal dialysis to hemodialysis." The medical terms roll off my tongue with an ease born of years of dealing with kidney issues. It's a language I never wanted to become fluent in, yet here I am, practically bilingual in the dialect of renal failure.

I pause, considering how to explain this to my kids who might one day watch this video. The thought of them possibly viewing this after I'm gone sends a pang through my heart, but I push through it. "Peritoneal dialysis is where they take fluids out of your stomach and clean them, but my body has changed so much in the past six weeks that I need to go with hemodialysis, which is where they filter your blood."

As I speak, I'm acutely aware of how my body feels – the heaviness in my limbs, the persistent ache in my lower back, the slight shortness of breath that comes with even minimal exertion. These are the physical manifestations of my kidneys' failure, the outward signs of the battle raging inside me.

The memory of my previous experience with hemodialysis in 2012 surfaces, bringing with it a mix of emotions. "I've done hemodialysis before, back when I had my first kidney transplant in 2012. It wasn't the best experience because the fistula in my left arm never worked properly."

I remember the frustration of those days – the long hours hooked up to the dialysis machine, the constant worry about infection, the way my life revolved around treatment schedules. It wasn't an easy time, but I got through it. The memory gives me a glimmer of hope – I've faced this before, I can face it again.

I shift in the chair, feeling the fatigue that seems to have seeped into my very bones. "So, for the next few weeks, I'll be doing hemodialysis through a neck port, or a chest port, probably. I'll have to keep it clean, but I'm not too worried about that."

A wry smile crosses my face as I remember my previous ordeal. "Back in 2012, I had to wait six weeks for a kidney with a chest port. I did everything I could to keep it clean during that time." I pause, correcting myself, "Actually, it was more like six months, but that's what's going on today."

As I finish speaking, I'm struck by the reality of what lies ahead. More procedures, more waiting, more uncertainty. But also, perhaps, a chance at life renewed. The monochrome world around me seems a little less bleak as I cling to that hope.

I turn off the recording and lean back in the chair, exhausted by even this small effort. Outside my room, I can hear the bustle of the hospital – nurses chatting, carts being wheeled down the corridor, the distant ding of an elevator. Life goes on, even here in this place of sickness and healing.

My thoughts turn to the long road ahead. Dialysis, possibly for months. The search for a donor kidney. The transplant itself, if I'm lucky enough to receive one. Recovery. It's a daunting journey, one that I'm not sure I have the strength for. But then I think of my family, my friends, all the people waiting for me to come home. Their love and support flow through me, bolstering my resolve.

I may be seeing the world in black and white right now, but I hold onto the promise of color returning to my life. Each day, each treatment, is a step towards that goal. As I settle in for whatever comes next, I make a silent promise to myself: I will fight. I will endure. I will see color again.

Chapter 4: The Procedure

The recovery room is dimly lit, a stark contrast to the harsh fluorescents of the main hospital areas. The soft lighting is a small mercy, easy on my tired eyes and aching head. I'm laid out in a hospital bed, the gown draped awkwardly over my chest, leaving my shoulders exposed to the cool air. The thin fabric does little to ward off the chill, and I find myself longing for the comfort of my hoodie.

The soft beeping of monitors provides a constant reminder of where I am and why I'm here. Each beep feels like a countdown, though to what, I'm not sure. Recovery? Further complications? The uncertainty is almost as uncomfortable as the physical discomfort.

I can feel the changes in my body acutely. My face feels even puffier than before, stretched and uncomfortable. When I gingerly reach up to touch my cheek, my fingers sink into the swollen flesh more than I expect. It's as if I'm wearing a mask of my own face, but one that doesn't quite fit right.

There's a fresh wound on my neck, swollen and tender, a new addition to the map of scars that tell the story of my medical journey. I can feel the bandage pulling at my skin with every slight movement. It's a constant, nagging sensation that makes it impossible to forget why I'm here, even for a moment.

The procedure itself is still vivid in my mind, despite the lingering effects of the anesthesia. I remember the cold antiseptic on my skin, the pressure of the surgeon's hands, the unsettling sensation of things happening to my body that I couldn't quite feel but was still somehow aware of.

When I speak, my voice comes out as a gravelly whisper, barely recognizable to my own ears. "Just got the catheter," I rasp, wincing slightly at the memory. "It's a little more intense than I remember."

I pause, gathering my thoughts through the fog of post-procedure discomfort. The words come slowly, each one requiring effort to push past my dry lips. "Because I'm normally not on the twilight anesthesia, which just means they push you around a bit, but you can still feel and hear everything that's going on."

The experience replays in my mind, vivid despite the anesthesia. I can still hear the murmur of the surgical team's voices, the clinking of instruments, the steady beep of the heart monitor. It's a sensory memory that I suspect will stay with me for a long time.

"They started operating on my right side, but there was too much scarring there, so they decided to put it on the left instead." I remember the moment of confusion, the sudden change of plans. It's a stark reminder of how my body has been through this before, how it bears the marks of past battles.

I try to shift in the bed, immediately regretting the movement. Pain lances through my neck and shoulder, causing me to inhale sharply. "But now, I feel like my body is like a stack of bricks. I'm not sure how that happened, but it's not fun."

As I lie there, feeling every ache and pain, I'm struck by the fragility of my situation. Each procedure, each day, feels like a step into unknown territory. The black and white world around me seems to pulse with each beep of the monitors, a visual representation of the binary nature of my current existence: progress or setback, life or death.

But even in this stark, colorless landscape, I find myself searching for shades of grey – small victories, moments of comfort, the unwavering support of my loved ones. It's these nuances that I cling to, that give me the strength to face whatever comes next in this journey.

I close my eyes, trying to find a comfortable position. The pillow feels too flat, the sheets too scratchy. Everything is a reminder that I'm not at home, that I'm in a place of healing but also of sickness. The smell of disinfectant tickles my nose, mingling with the metallic scent that seems to cling to me after the procedure.

My thoughts drift to my family. Are they worried? Have they been updated about the procedure? I make a mental note to ask the nurse if I can make a call once I feel a bit more human. The thought of hearing their voices, of reassuring them (and myself) that I'm okay, gives me a small burst of energy.

As I lie in the recovery room, caught between the lingering effects of anesthesia and the gradual return to full awareness, I find myself taking stock. This catheter, this new addition to my body, is both a lifeline and a tether. It's a reminder of my illness, yes, but also a path to treatment, to getting better.

I've been here before, I remind myself. I've faced dialysis and transplants and all the complications that come with them. I've seen the other side of this, felt the joy of recovery, of reclaiming my life. That memory, that knowledge, is a comfort. It's a light in the monochrome world I'm currently inhabiting.

The nurse comes in to check on me, her movements efficient but gentle. She asks about my pain level, adjusts my IV, makes a note on my chart. Her presence is reassuring, a reminder that I'm not alone in this sterile, beeping room.

As she leaves, I settle back into the pillows. The procedure is over. The catheter is in place. It's not comfortable, it's not pleasant, but it's necessary. It's a step forward on this journey, a journey I'm determined to see through to the end.

The rhythmic beeping of the monitors gradually fades into the background as exhaustion takes over. My last thoughts before drifting off to sleep are of color – of the vibrant world waiting for me beyond these hospital walls, of the life I'm fighting to return to. In this moment, on this day, in this recovery room, I make a silent promise to myself: I will see those colors again.

Chapter 5: Visitors and Progress

The monotony of the hospital room is suddenly broken by a splash of color - a stuffed lion, its mane a vibrant gold against the stark white sheets. I can't help but smile as I hold it, feeling a childlike comfort from its soft fur against my hands.

"Things aren't all bad, though," I say to the camera, my voice stronger than it's been in days. "I've got my first visitor, and his name is Lion. He's a lion, of course, and he's from the Sticking Place. So, I can stick my courage to it."

The Shakespeare reference brings a warmth to my chest, a reminder of happier times on stage. "He was brought to me by one of my favorite castmates ever. Go ahead and introduce yourself," I say, turning the camera to my visitor.

Sharron, a whirlwind of energy in her early 50s, beams at the camera. "Hi, it's me, Sharron! Marc is looking mighty fit and fabulous these days!" Her enthusiasm is infectious, and I find myself sitting up a little straighter. "He's gonna do great once this dialysis thing gets going. In just a couple of hours, he'll be all set."

As Sharron continues, encouraging people to send texts and organizing a meal train, I'm struck by her efficiency. It's exactly what I need right now - someone to take charge when I'm feeling so powerless.

"Sharron, I just want to thank you so much for being here," I say, my gratitude overwhelming me for a moment. "My wife Teri is diagnosed with pneumonia and it just happened like yesterday so we're just kind of in a weird place."

I pause, gathering my thoughts. "Sharron is here being a boss, doing her upper-class white lady duties, asking questions and getting everyone in gear. I'm like, 'Wow, I didn't even think to ask that.' But thank you so much, Sharron, I really appreciate it."

"I love you, Marc," Sharron says, her eyes shining with sincerity.

"Love you too. Alright, thanks," I respond, feeling a lump in my throat. These moments of connection, of love from my friends, are what keep me going through the difficult days.

Suddenly, Sharron's attention is drawn to my feet. "So, if you've ever seen Marc's feet they are in fact extra large, however they're not usually quite this swollen, look at this swelling!"

I laugh nervously, uncomfortable with the attention on my swollen limbs but appreciating Sharron's attempt to lighten the mood.

"It's kind of like... um... it's like walking like a stone giant so it's kind of painful," I explain, trying to put words to the strange sensation. "But hopefully the dialysis will start today and it will start to take that down. I'm really appreciative of all the work everybody's doing to help me now. But, that's the feets!"

As Sharron leaves, I'm left alone with my thoughts and the stuffed lion. The room feels emptier without her vibrant presence, but I'm buoyed by the visit. It's a reminder that I'm not alone in this fight, that there are people out there rooting for me.

I settle back against the pillows, clutching the lion to my chest. The beeping of the monitors fades into the background as I close my eyes, allowing myself a moment of rest. Tomorrow will bring more challenges, more dialysis, more uncertainty. But for now, I have this moment of peace, this token of love from a friend, and the knowledge that I'm not facing this alone.

As I drift off to sleep, I make a mental note to ask the nurse about starting dialysis. The sooner we start, the sooner I can begin to feel like myself again. The sooner I can return to the colorful world that Sharron brought a glimpse of into my monochrome hospital room.

The next day brings an unexpected visitor - Dr. Ray, my nephrologist. I've been dozing, the camera forgotten and still recording, when his voice pulls me back to consciousness.

"I think what we need to do is kind of slowly get you stabilized and I also-" Dr. Ray is saying as I blink awake.

"Was that all evident by the numbers that we drew when I came here?" I interrupt, my mind struggling to catch up with the conversation.

Dr. Ray nods, his expression serious. "That's right, hemoglobin is really low and you're not able to lay completely flat."

I shift in the bed, realizing that I am indeed propped up on several pillows. "Yeah it's much better now, I feel," I say, surprised by the improvement I hadn't noticed until now.

"And also, you know, the heart silhouette is enlarged so I told the medical physician to check an echocardiogram to see if there's any fluid around the heart," Dr. Ray continues.

His words hit me like a punch to the gut. Heart problems on top of everything else? I feel a wave of guilt wash over me.

"Am I... was I not making like, I feel like I was sending messages when I needed to but I feel like maybe I was letting things get too out of control because I figured I could still take care of it..." The words tumble out of me in a rush. "Are we here because I thought I could just ride my bike forever and then everything would be good? That's basically it?"

Dr. Ray's expression softens. "I told you, right, you're going to be fine and then all of a sudden it's going to drop off."

His words bring back memories of previous conversations, warnings I had brushed aside in my determination to maintain normalcy. "Cause I feel like in the last month everything just collapsed. Nothing even makes sense now. It's like I'm not even the same person.... I'm sorry for not listening to you then."

"It's okay, it's okay," Dr. Ray reassures me, his voice gentle. "The problem... All these things are fixable. It's just that the route is going to be a little different from the route we initially planned because of what's going on with your health. But we're eventually going to get you to Peritoneal Dialysis."

I nod, clinging to his words like a lifeline. "Alright. Alright."

"We're going to get you dialyzed today for two hours, three hours tomorrow, and then four hours the day after that," Dr. Ray explains.

As he leaves, I'm left with a mix of emotions - relief that there's a plan, guilt for not heeding earlier warnings, fear of what's to come, but also a glimmer of hope. The path ahead is different than what we'd planned, but there is a path. And for now, that has to be enough.

Chapter 6: Small Victories

The next morning, I wake up feeling... different. Not better, exactly, but less worse. It's a subtle shift, but after weeks of steady decline, even this small improvement feels monumental.

I manage to move from the bed to one of the room chairs, the effort leaving me breathless but accomplished. Settling into the chair, I pick up my phone to record another update for my friends and kids.

"Here's another update," I begin, my voice stronger than it's been in days. "I had my port installed yesterday and I have a second round of dialysis coming up today. I feel a lot better... I've lost about six... about six pounds of water."

The weight loss, though modest, feels like a victory. It's tangible proof that the treatments are working, that my body is fighting back against the flood of toxins.

"So I'm on my mission towards health," I continue, allowing a note of optimism to creep into my voice. "Um, long term, I don't want to stick with this port up here I want to have one in my stomach but I've got to go through a couple of steps first to make sure that I'm not still bleeding internally..."

I pause, considering how to phrase the next part. "I was able to eat a lot of food today mostly fruit 'cause when I tried to eat bread my throat was like-" I make an exaggerated puking sound, laughing a little at my own joke. "But I haven't thrown up today and I think my second dialysis will be coming soon."

As I finish the update, thanking those who have visited, I'm struck by how much better I feel just for having spoken, for having connected with the outside world. It's a reminder that healing isn't just physical - it's emotional and social too.

Later that day, my room is transformed by the arrival of two very special visitors - my mother, Mary George, and my friend Babs. Their presence brings color back into my monochrome world, filling the sterile hospital room with warmth and love.

"My day is getting really great because I have one of my favorite people, Babs George. And my mother, Mary George, is here to visit me," I say to the camera, unable to keep the joy from my voice.

Babs, despite being a classically trained actor, seems nervous in front of the phone camera. "That's all. Hi. We love our Marc. Oh and we're very, we're very, I don't know, oh-" she stumbles over her words, and I can't help but find it endearing.

"It's all good, Babs," I reassure her, before turning to my mother. "Mom, anything to say?"

My mother's face lights up as she speaks. "Yesterday when I saw you? I was totally blown away by how much better you look today!" Her words fill me with a mixture of hope and concern - how bad must I have looked yesterday? "Honestly, when I first saw you, I was a bit hesitant to say anything because your face was so swollen and puffy. I mean, I drove all the way from the valley to see you, and seeing you in that state was a bit of a shock. But I held back and didn't say anything at the time."

Her honesty is both touching and sobering. I knew I was in bad shape, but hearing it from my mother drives home just how serious my condition was - and still is.

"But today, it's awesome to see you laughing and making videos!" she continues, her smile wide and genuine. "It's a testament to how far you've come!"

Her words buoy me, reminding me of the progress I've made. Even if I'm not out of the woods yet, I'm moving in the right direction.

As the days progress, I find myself settling into a routine of dialysis and recovery. After my second round of treatment, I feel well enough to walk around the room and deliver another update.

Standing in front of the mirror, I'm struck by how much more like myself I look and sound. "One of the good things about dialysis is that it clears the toxins from your blood," I explain to the camera. "I'm able to walk around now and my voice sounds a little bit more like it used to."

I go on to explain about uremia and the fluid buildup in my body. "I've got about maybe 20 lbs. of fluid which is overweight and it was about 30 that I gained in about a week and a half but after two days of treatment I feel pretty good."

As I speak, I'm acutely aware of the long road ahead. "The thing is that this is going to have to be a permanent solution. It's not a real permanent solution. The real permanent solution is getting a kidney transplant at some point but for now this is going to keep me alive."

The reality of my situation settles over me like a weight. This is my life now - dialysis, hospital visits, the constant quest for a donor kidney. But as I look at myself in the mirror, I see not just the illness, but the fight. I see a man who's not giving up, who's surrounded by love and support, who's taking each day as it comes.

Yes, the world is still largely black and white. But there are hints of color creeping in - the gold of the stuffed lion, the warmth in my mother's smile, the hope in my own eyes reflected back at me. And for now, that's enough to keep me going.

My next dialysis session stretches out before me - four long hours tethered to a machine. As I settle in for the treatment, I'm joined by a small group of visitors: my dialysis nurse, my mother, and my friends Alex and Laura.

"4 hours today? You told me not to get bored," I say to the nurse, trying to inject some humor into the situation.

As Alex and Laura discuss vaccinations in the background, I clumsily try to include them in my ongoing documentation of this journey. "I already have four. I got four or five but I'm here right now in the middle of my third dialysis treatment and I've got... I've got, well I've got my mother, hey Mom, I've got Alex Alford from Austin Shakespeare and I've got Laura as well. You guys can talk a little bit more about yourself or just what you are doing here."

Alex steps forward, his face kind. "Hi everybody. Marc looks great and he's sounding great, he's doing really well."

"Awesome, thank you," I respond, touched by his positivity.

Laura chimes in, "Absolutely, we're just happy to be here."

Their presence, their willingness to sit with me through this long process, fills me with gratitude. Even as the dialysis machine hums and beeps, even as I feel the pull of toxins leaving my body, I'm reminded that I'm not alone in this fight.

As the session continues, I find myself reflecting on the journey so far. The fear and uncertainty of those first days in the hospital seem distant now, replaced by a cautious optimism. Yes, there's still a long road ahead. Yes, there will be more challenges to face. But with each treatment, with each visitor, with each small victory, I feel myself growing stronger.

The world may still be largely monochrome, but the colors are slowly, surely, beginning to return. And I'm determined to see them all again, in their full vibrant glory.

Chapter 7: The Road Ahead

The familiar face of Dr. Ray brings a sense of comfort as he enters my hospital room. Despite the seriousness of my condition, seeing him reminds me that I'm in capable hands. I fumble for my phone, determined to document this conversation for my own records and for my family.

"This is my doctor, Dr. Ray," I say to the camera, my voice stronger than it's been in days. "He's been guiding me through this journey for a few years now, and he's just giving me an update about where we are in my third or fourth day here, I'm not sure, of the hospital."

Dr. Ray nods, his expression a mix of concern and reassurance. "Yeah, you came here on Thursday."

"Correct. Thursday evening," I confirm, the days blurring together in my mind. It feels like I've been here for weeks, not days.

Dr. Ray leans in, his eyes searching my face. "How are you feeling, Marc?"

I take a moment to assess myself. The improvement, while not complete, is significant. "I feel worlds better physically. I feel worlds better. I was-"

"How's the nausea?" Dr. Ray interrupts, getting straight to the point.

"The nausea has gone completely," I say, realizing it as I speak. It's a small victory, but it feels monumental. "I haven't thrown up in... in at least two days. At least, well, I guess the second day is the first... the last day I threw up."

We continue through a checklist of symptoms - appetite (improved), breathing (better, though my voice is still affected), and overall condition. As we talk, I can feel the weight of worry lifting slightly from my shoulders. I'm not out of the woods, not by a long shot, but I'm better than I was. It's progress.

The conversation shifts to more serious matters - my ongoing treatment plan. Dr. Ray explains the hesitation of the vascular surgeon to insert a catheter right away, the need for more dialysis to reduce fluid retention, and the concerns about my blood pressure.

As he speaks, my mind races ahead. "Now, that brings me to my next question," I interject, unable to contain my worry. "Couple questions: what is the long-term plan to stop me from internal bleeding? Because I keep losing blood, and if it's internal bleeding, what's the long-term plan for that?"

Dr. Ray's response is measured, reminding me of previous tests and the need for further investigation. We discuss the possibility of a colonoscopy, the use of Epogen therapy to boost my blood count, and the complexities of finding the source of the bleeding.

As we talk, I can feel my mother's presence in the room, even though she's not here. Her worried face floats in my mind, spurring me to ask more questions. "I'm asking all these questions because these are all the questions my mother keeps asking," I explain to Dr. Ray.

We move on to discuss outpatient dialysis options. The decision of where to continue my treatment weighs heavily on me. Dr. Ray presents the options, emphasizing that the choice is mine. I can feel the importance of this decision - it's not just about logistics, it's about the course of my treatment, potentially for months to come.

"Then I'll choose to continue to be under your care," I decide, "because you are familiar with my previous case." The relief on Dr. Ray's face is palpable, and I know I've made the right choice.

Our conversation takes an unexpected turn when I mention a potential living donor. Dr. Ray's surprise is evident, and we dive into the complexities of the transplant process. It's a maze of ethical considerations, medical evaluations, and bureaucratic procedures.

"I think there are a lot of steps here we need to figure out," Dr. Ray says, tempering my excitement with reality. We discuss the need for me to be officially listed for a transplant, the various tests and evaluations required, and the time frame we're looking at.

"I'm thinking if everybody and everything goes perfectly according to plan, it might take about 3 months," Dr. Ray estimates. It's longer than I'd hoped, but shorter than I'd feared. A timeline I can work with.

As our conversation winds down, I'm filled with a mix of emotions - hope for the progress I've made, anxiety about the long road ahead, gratitude for Dr. Ray's care and guidance.

"Alright. Well, I think you answered just about all my questions. I appreciate your help. Thanks a lot, doc," I say, my voice thick with emotion.

"Of course," Dr. Ray responds, his tone warm.

"You saved my life," I add, the weight of those words hitting me as I say them.

"You bet. Anytime. Definitely," Dr. Ray replies, his modesty evident.

As Dr. Ray leaves, I'm left alone with my thoughts. The room feels different somehow - still stark and clinical, but filled with possibility. The path ahead is long and uncertain, but for the first time in days, I feel like I can see it stretching out before me.

I lean back against my pillows, exhausted but oddly invigorated. The world around me is still largely monochrome, but there are hints of color creeping in at the edges. The warm brown of Dr. Ray's eyes, the soft blue of the sky visible through my window, the vibrant red of hope blossoming in my chest.

There's still so much to do, so many hurdles to overcome. But I'm not alone in this fight. I have Dr. Ray, my family, my friends, and my own determination. As I close my eyes, allowing myself to rest, I make a silent promise to myself: I will walk this path, no matter how difficult. I will see this through. I will find my way back to the full spectrum of life, one step at a time.

Chapter 8: Progress and Preparations

Day 5 dawns, and I find myself settling into a strange new routine in the hospital. The stark white walls have become familiar, the beeping of machines a constant backdrop to my thoughts. I reach for my phone, determined to keep my friends and family updated on my progress.

"Another update for day five," I begin, my voice stronger than it's been in days. "I had a long chat with my doctor about my health. We decided I'd get two more dialysis treatments while I'm still here. These treatments will help clean my blood and make me feel better overall."

As I speak, I can feel the difference in my body. The heaviness that had weighed me down just days ago is lifting, replaced by a cautious optimism. "Compared to how I was five days ago, I feel a whole lot better," I continue. "The dialysis treatments have helped get rid of the toxins and extra fluid in my body, and I'm actually hungry again!"

The return of appetite feels like a small miracle. I remember the days when the thought of food turned my stomach, when even water was a challenge to keep down. Now, I find myself looking forward to meal times, a simple pleasure I'd nearly forgotten.

"I'm thankful for the care and support I've gotten from the hospital staff, and I'm sure I'll keep getting better," I conclude, meaning every word. The nurses, doctors, and staff have become a sort of surrogate family, their care and dedication a lifeline in this sterile environment.

As night falls, a new challenge presents itself. I've been scheduled for a colonoscopy, a crucial step in my treatment plan. The procedure itself doesn't worry me – it's the preparation that's daunting.

"Here's the mission," I explain to my phone camera, a hint of humor in my voice despite the late hour. "I have until midnight. It is now 10:20 because I had a round of dialysis that was done a little bit late today. I've got to drink this gallon-shaped container of some kind of fluid."

The container looms large on my bedside table, a formidable opponent in the quiet of the night. But I'm not facing this challenge alone. My wife Teri has arrived, a welcome sight after days of separation.

"My wife Teri has made it here thanks to some very kind help and loaner vehicles," I say, gratitude evident in my voice. Her presence is a comfort, a reminder of the life waiting for me beyond these hospital walls.

As I prepare for the long night ahead, I'm buoyed by another reminder of the support system surrounding me. "Want to thank a group of my college friends," I say, gesturing to a new hat perched on my head. "We call ourselves the Core Black Folk meeting. We have online meetings, and they sent me one of these two nice hats because they knew that I was cold all the time."

The hat is more than just warmth – it's a tangible connection to my friends, to the world outside. As I settle in for the night, steeling myself for the task ahead, I'm filled with a mix of emotions. Apprehension about the procedure, yes, but also hope. Hope that this colonoscopy will provide answers, will be another step on the path to recovery.

The night stretches long before me, but I'm no longer daunted. I've faced worse in the past week, and I know I can face this too. One sip at a time, one hour at a time, I'll make it through. And tomorrow, hopefully, we'll have more answers, more progress to celebrate.

As I reach for the first cup of the prep solution, I take a deep breath. This is just another hurdle to overcome, another step on the journey back to health. With Teri by my side and the support of friends near and far, I know I can do this. I have to do this. It's all part of the fight to reclaim my life, to see the world in full color once again.

Day 7 arrives, marking a full week since my admission to the hospital. The change in my condition is dramatic, and I'm eager to share the good news with my friends and family.

"Good morning. Here's my day seven update," I begin, barely able to contain my excitement. "It is Wednesday, and I got here Wednesday a week ago. I've lost about anywhere between 25 and 30 lbs. They haven't really put me back on the scale, but I feel totally different."

As I speak, I'm struck by how much stronger my voice sounds. "My voice, as you can tell, is back to pretty... very close to what it was before I started this. The same voice I used to book a lot of acting jobs."

The return of my voice feels like reclaiming a part of myself. It's more than just a physical improvement – it's a connection to my identity, to the career I love.

"I'm not in pain," I continue, marveling at the realization. "My feet are normal, they're not swollen. My legs are normal again." Each of these improvements feels like a small victory, steps towards reclaiming my health and my life.

I outline the plan for the day – one last in-hospital dialysis treatment, then release in the afternoon. The future is starting to take shape, with plans for a PD catheter insertion the next day. "That's a great goal that we're able to shorten the time on," I say, feeling a surge of optimism.

As I recount the results of yesterday's colonoscopy and endoscopy, I'm relieved to report that no bleeding was found. There's one more test on the horizon – a small scope that will travel through my digestive system. "It reminds me of that 80s movie 'Inner Space'," I joke, finding humor even in these medical procedures.

But as I continue talking, I notice my voice starting to falter slightly. It's a reminder that recovery is a process, that there will be good days and bad. "As I start to book gigs again, voice-over gigs, I'll make sure to have apple juice or water in the booth with me," I muse, already planning for the future.

The overwhelming gratitude I feel comes pouring out as I conclude my update. "I can't thank you guys enough, the people who have supported my family and I throughout this ordeal," I say, my voice thick with emotion. "I came in here a week ago on death's door, literally on that door, and the first weekend was not looking good at all. And then when I asked for help, you guys came through in an unbelievable, truly unbelievable fashion."

As I end the recording, I'm filled with a sense of hope and determination. The road ahead is still long, but I'm no longer walking it alone. With the support of my medical team, my family, and my friends, I know I can face whatever challenges lie ahead. The world is slowly regaining its color, and I'm ready to embrace it fully.

Chapter 9: New Beginnings and Harsh Realities

Day 8 arrives, bringing with it unexpected changes to the plan. I've learned over the past week that flexibility is key in this journey, and today is no exception.

"I'm going to give you one more update," I begin, settling into what has become a familiar routine. "As we've often seen in the last week, plans change, and they did yesterday, not in a bad way. Today is day eight. I'm here on Thursday. I arrived here last Wednesday. It's 8 days."

I explain the change in plans – staying an extra night for observation instead of being discharged. It's a small adjustment, but one that I hope will lead to better outcomes. "Sorry that I got everybody's hopes up, but I did not go home yesterday. I've been here one more day," I say, a hint of apology in my voice.

Despite the extended stay, my spirits are high. "It's funny that I have become a local celebrity here," I share, unable to keep the amusement from my voice. "Everybody is excited to learn that I'm an actor and I've played in plays around town. They come and ask me about stuff. That's lifting my spirits, it's really fun."

The attention is a welcome distraction from the medical procedures ahead. I detail the changes to my treatment plan – going straight to peritoneal dialysis after the catheter placement instead of two more weeks of hemodialysis. It's a faster transition than expected, but one I'm eager to embrace.

"Wish me luck and one more day, or at least a couple more hours before I get surgery," I say, a mix of anticipation and nervousness in my voice. The support I've received continues to overwhelm me, and I make sure to acknowledge it. "I want to send another thank you out to the people who have already teamed up to watch me at home because I've got a few people that are watching me at home today as Teri slowly returns back to work with her pneumonia subsiding."

As I end the update, I'm filled with a sense of anticipation. Tomorrow brings new challenges – surgery, the start of training for home dialysis – but also new possibilities. It's another step towards reclaiming my life, towards independence.

The world comes back into focus slowly, pain being the first sensation to register. I'm in a recovery room, the surgery to place my PD catheter complete. The stark fluorescent lights above me seem too bright, too harsh.

"Out of surgery," I manage to say weakly, my voice barely above a whisper. "My stomach is killing me."

The pain is intense, radiating from the site of the new catheter. It's a sharp reminder of the physical toll this journey is taking on my body. But beneath the pain, there's a glimmer of hope. This catheter is a key to my future independence, a tool that will allow me to manage my dialysis from home.

As I lie there, trying to breathe through the discomfort, I'm struck by the absence of pain medication. I wonder, not for the first time, if my race plays a role in this oversight. As a Black man, I'm acutely aware of the disparities in healthcare, particularly when it comes to pain management. The thought sends a chill through me, colder than the sterile air of the recovery room.

The next thing I know, I'm being wheeled out of the hospital. The transition is abrupt – one moment in the cocoon of hospital care, the next facing the outside world again. My friend Shannon is there to drive me home, her car a welcome sight after days of sterile hospital surroundings.

"Oh, right here to my messy car," Shannon says apologetically.

"That's all good, Shannon," I reassure her, grateful for her help. "Just say 'what's up' to the camera."

Shannon's simple "Hi" to the camera is a bridge between my hospital stay and the return to normal life. As I'm helped into her car, I'm struck by how different everything looks. The world seems brighter, more vivid, despite the lingering effects of the surgery and the nagging pain that still hasn't been addressed.

The next morning arrives all too quickly. It's time for my first peritoneal dialysis training class, and despite the lingering pain from surgery, I'm determined to face this new challenge head-on.

"Alright, we're on our way to our first peritoneal dialysis class this morning," I say to the camera as Teri drives us. The familiar routine of documenting my journey helps calm my nerves. "I hope you can hear from my voice and my face that after about 8 days, I feel a lot better, thanks to the hemodialysis that I already had. I'm really looking forward to the progress I'm going to continue to make with the peritoneal dialysis."

I turn to Teri, concern for her health mixing with gratitude for her unwavering support. "I'm here with Teri, who's hopefully feeling a little bit better from her pneumonia. How you feeling, baby?"

Teri's tired "Tired" speaks volumes about the toll this ordeal has taken on her as well. "Yes, Teri's been a superhero this week," I say, wanting to acknowledge her efforts. "Really helping me out even from home, taking care of things and helping to coordinate with other people to come and watch me in the hospital or bring gifts or food."

The training itself is a blur of information and pain. My nurse is excellent, patient and thorough, but the lingering surgical pain makes it hard to focus. Teri, true to form, takes copious notes, a fact I'm immensely grateful for.

As we drive home, the lack of post-surgical pain medication becomes a pressing issue. "My surgeon didn't prescribe any pain medicine after the surgery yesterday," I explain, frustration creeping into my voice. "Which was surprising to myself, to the nurses on call, to just about everybody I've talked to."

The bureaucratic maze of trying to get pain relief is maddening. Calls to the surgeon's office, to the hospital, to the pharmacy – all seem to lead nowhere. As I recount the difficulties, I'm struck by a larger pattern I've noticed during my hospital stay.

"But it's part of a larger pattern because when I was in the hospital, I dealt with pain just about every day. Sincere, real pain, different pains for different reasons," I say, the words coming out in a rush. "Most times I was talked to as if I wasn't experiencing what I was experiencing, or I was given an assurance that 'yes, I understand that you're having pain,' and then given no pain medicine."

The frustration and disappointment are palpable in my voice as I conclude, "I shouldn't have to look like my care provider to get the care that I need."

As these words leave my mouth, their full weight hits me. I shouldn't have to look like my care provider – but the reality is, in many cases, I don't. As a Black man in America, I'm all too aware of the disparities in healthcare. Studies have shown that Black patients are systematically undertreated for pain, their symptoms often dismissed or minimized.

I think about the documented cases of medical professionals, including doctors, being trained to believe that Black people don't feel pain as acutely as others. It's a belief rooted in centuries of racist pseudoscience, yet its effects are still felt today, in hospitals across the country. I think about Serena Williams, one of the most recognized athletes in the world, being ignored when she was in distress during childbirth. If it can happen to her, what chance do ordinary Black men and women have?

The realization sits heavily in my chest, alongside the physical pain from the surgery. This journey isn't just about my personal battle with kidney disease – it's about a larger fight. A fight for equitable healthcare, for the right to be heard and believed when we say we're in pain. A fight for reform in all aspects of healthcare – insurance, patient advocacy, addressing the glaring disparities that persist despite advances in medical science.

As we pull into our driveway, I'm hit by a wave of conflicting emotions. Joy at being home, excitement about the new dialysis regimen, frustration at the pain and the difficulties in getting it addressed, and an overwhelming sense of purpose. This experience, as challenging as it is, has opened my eyes to the broader issues at play. I realize that my story, my journey, can be a vehicle for change.

I step out of the car, wincing at the pain but determined. This is just the beginning of a new phase in my journey. There will be challenges ahead – learning the intricacies of home dialysis, managing my health, hopefully moving towards a transplant. But now, I see a bigger picture. My fight isn't just for my own health – it's for everyone who has ever been dismissed, disbelieved, or undertreated because of the color of their skin.

As I walk into my house, I make a silent promise to myself. I will continue to document this journey, to speak out about my experiences, good and bad. I will use my voice – the same voice that's brought characters to life on stage and screen – to advocate for change. For healthcare reform, for patient rights, for equality in medical treatment.

The world is slowly regaining its color, but I see it now with new eyes. Eyes that are open to the injustices, the disparities, the work that still needs to be done. One step at a time, I'm reclaiming my life. But more than that, I'm committing to a larger cause. The journey continues, but now it's about more than just my recovery. It's about paving the way for a future where everyone, regardless of race, receives the care and respect they deserve in their most vulnerable moments.

Chapter 10: Family, Progress, and New Horizons

The doorbell chimes, its familiar sound cutting through the quiet of the house. My heart leaps – a mixture of excitement and nervousness. I've been looking forward to this visit, but it's also a stark reminder of how much has changed. I grab my phone, determined to document this moment, and make my way to the door. Each step is still a bit labored, a reminder of my recent ordeal, but I'm moving better than I have in weeks.

As I open the door, I'm greeted by the sight of Eric, my son, and Angela, his mother. The rush of emotion is overwhelming – joy at seeing them, pride at how much Eric has grown, and a tinge of sadness that my other son couldn't make it. It's a bittersweet cocktail of feelings that I'm learning to navigate in this new chapter of my life.

"What's going on! Come on in. It's alright, come on in," I say, trying to infuse my voice with as much warmth and normalcy as possible. "Did Marc not want to come?"

Angela explains that he was still asleep, and Eric chimes in about their difficulty waking him. I nod, understanding the challenges of rousing a teenager. There's a moment of awkwardness – we're all acutely aware of the time that's passed, the events that have transpired. I'm searching for words to bridge the gap when I notice a delivery person at the door. Perfect timing, a welcome distraction.

After thanking the delivery person, I turn back to Eric and Angela, gesturing to my phone. "Alright, don't mind the camera. I'm just putting some stuff together for a... I don't know what it's going to be, maybe a short film, maybe a documentary." The uncertainty in my voice reflects my broader feelings – I'm not quite sure where this journey is taking me, but I feel compelled to document it.

I study Eric, marveling at how much he's grown. It's a cliché, but it's true – they really do grow up so fast, especially when health issues force you to miss chunks of time. "Are you still feeling some symptoms, Eric?" I ask, concerned about his recent illness. The worry in my voice is palpable – after my own health scare, I find myself hyper-aware of any sign of illness in my loved ones.

"No, I haven't felt any since last week," he assures me. His voice, deeper than I remember, is another reminder of the passage of time.

"Good Lord, you've gotten even taller," I can't help but exclaim. "Take a picture of us." As we pose for the photo, I'm struck by the physical changes in my son. "Okay, look, after all this... wow, he has got to be 6 foot 6." Pride swells in my chest, mingled with a touch of wistfulness for the time I've missed. I find myself wondering how many growth spurts I've missed, how many milestones have passed while I was fighting my own battles.

We chat about school, basketball, and his upcoming plans. The conversation feels both familiar and strange – I'm trying to reconnect, to be the involved father I want to be, while also navigating the new reality of my health situation. When he mentions going to a Travis Scott concert, I feel a pang of parental worry. "Be careful," I caution, remembering the tragedy at Scott's last concert. It's a delicate balance – wanting to protect him while also letting him live his life.

As our conversation winds down, I'm filled with a complex mix of emotions. Joy at seeing my son, gratitude for this moment of normalcy amidst my health struggles, and a renewed determination to be there for more moments like these in the future. There's also a lingering sadness – for the time lost, for the strain my illness has put on our relationship. But overwhelmingly, there's hope. Hope that we can rebuild, strengthen our bond, and create new memories together.

The visit ends all too soon, and as I watch Eric and Angela drive away, I'm hit with a wave of emotion. I close the door and lean against it, taking a deep breath. This visit has reinforced my resolve to fight, to get healthy, to be there for my children. It's not just about surviving anymore – it's about living, about being present for these precious moments with my family.

The scene shifts to the dialysis clinic, where Marta, my training nurse, is showing Teri and me how to set up the machine. The room is filled with the hum of medical equipment, a sound that's become all too familiar in recent weeks. The antiseptic smell of the clinic is a constant reminder of the gravity of my situation, but today, it's tinged with a sense of possibility.

"A new machine, right when you get yours, is going to ask us for the activation code," Marta explains, her voice patient and reassuring. As she continues detailing the process, I feel a strange mix of excitement and trepidation. This machine, with its tubes and dials and digital readouts, is my lifeline. It's daunting, yes, but it's also my ticket to more independence, a way to reclaim some control over my life and health.

I glance at Teri, seeing the concentration on her face as she takes notes. Her dedication moves me – she's been my rock through all of this, and here she is, learning alongside me, ready to support me in this new phase of our life together. I reach out and squeeze her hand, a silent thank you for everything she's done and continues to do.

As Marta goes through the steps, I try to absorb every detail. It's overwhelming – there's so much to remember, so many potential points of failure. But I'm determined to master this. I have to. This knowledge, this ability to manage my own care, is crucial to maintaining some semblance of a normal life.

"Other than that, you will not need it, alright?" Marta concludes, referring to the activation code. "I'm going to give you a website where this is all together." Her confidence in our ability to handle this is reassuring, but I can't help but feel the weight of responsibility settling on my shoulders. This isn't just about following instructions – it's about keeping myself alive, day after day.

Later, as I sit in the training chair, I take a moment to reflect on the recent changes in my life. The clinic is quiet, the only sounds the soft beep of machines and the muffled voices of staff in the hallway. I pull out my phone, compelled to document this moment, to share my progress with those who have supported me through this ordeal.

"This is the view from my training chair," I say to the camera, panning around to show the medical equipment that now plays such a crucial role in my life. "Things are looking up. I left the hospital last Thursday night. I spent a weekend eating mostly strawberries and grapes, but I lost another 3 lbs. over the weekend even without taking dialysis. I feel great."

I pause, taking off my mask to speak more clearly. "I'll take this mask down just in case you can't hear me. Nobody else is in the room." The act of removing the mask, even briefly, feels liberating. It's a small thing, but it's a reminder of the progress I've made, of the increasing moments of normalcy in my life.

"I feel great," I continue, and I mean it. Compared to where I was just weeks ago, the improvement is remarkable. "I saw my youngest son yesterday, he's taller than ever, and I just got a call back from the transplant clinic. They're looking forward to moving forward with the evaluation in December. Maybe by the start of 2024, we can have a transplant in the works."

As I speak these words, I feel a surge of hope. The future, which seemed so bleak and uncertain not long ago, is now filled with possibility. The prospect of a transplant, of a life free from dialysis, seems within reach. It's not a guarantee, I know that, but it's a goal to work towards, a light at the end of this long, challenging tunnel.

"I really love that I already have a few people that are volunteering to get tested," I say, my voice thick with emotion. The generosity of these potential donors, some of whom I barely know, continues to amaze me. "This has been the trial of my life, and the support that you guys have given me has been overwhelming, but we're still not done yet."

As I sit there, surrounded by the trappings of my new reality – the dialysis machine, the medical charts, the antiseptic smell of the clinic – I'm struck by how far I've come. Just weeks ago, I was fighting for my life in a hospital bed. Now, I'm learning to manage my own care, looking forward to a potential transplant, reconnecting with my family. The journey has been brutal, marked by pain, fear, and uncertainty. But it's also been illuminating, showing me the depth of love and support I have in my life, revealing strengths I didn't know I possessed.

"I'm just glad that I had the presence of mind to be able to go to the hospital when I did, or I don't know what would have happened," I reflect, a shiver running through me at the thought of what might have been. "But thank you all for your support. Love you all. Thank you."

As I end the recording, I lean back in the chair, taking a deep breath. The path ahead is still long and uncertain, filled with challenges I can't yet foresee. But in this moment, in this sterile clinic that represents both my lifeline and my temporary prison, I feel a sense of peace. Whatever comes next, I know I'm not facing it alone. And that knowledge gives me the strength to face each day, each treatment, each hurdle with determination and hope.

Thanksgiving arrives, and with it, a profound sense of gratitude that I've never experienced before. The house is filled with the aroma of cooking food – a feast that, just weeks ago, I wasn't sure I'd be here to enjoy. Teri and I stand together in our living room, the warmth of the fireplace a stark contrast to the chill of the hospital rooms I've become so accustomed to.

I pick up my phone, feeling the need to share this moment, to express the overwhelming thankfulness that threatens to choke me up. Teri stands close, her presence a comfort and strength as always. We've been through so much together, and this moment feels like a milestone, a celebration of survival and love.

"Hey, good morning and Happy Thanksgiving to everybody," I begin, my arm around Teri. My voice is stronger than it's been in months, a fact that doesn't escape my notice. "Teri and I really want to wish you a very Happy Thanksgiving because two weeks ago I was in the hospital fighting for my life. Teri was fighting pneumonia, but within hours, you guys came through and showed us the kind of love and support that we couldn't even imagine that we had in this community, and that's what we're really thankful for this year."

As I speak, memories of those dark days in the hospital flood back – the pain, the fear, the uncertainty. But they're overshadowed by the recollection of the outpouring of support we received. Friends bringing food, offering rides, sending messages of encouragement. The nurse who went above and beyond to ensure my comfort. The doctors who fought tirelessly to save my life. The strangers who offered prayers and well-wishes. In those moments of crisis, we discovered the true depth of our community, and it's left me humbled and profoundly grateful.

"Teri wants to say hi," I say, turning the camera to my wife. Her smile, though tired, is radiant. She's been my rock through all of this, fighting her own battle with pneumonia while supporting me every step of the way. As she waves to the camera, I'm struck anew by her strength, her resilience, her unwavering love.

"We just are grateful for everything you've done for us so far and thankful for you as friends and family," I continue, my voice thick with emotion. This Thanksgiving feels different, more poignant than any before. Every breath is a gift, every moment with loved ones precious beyond measure.

As we conclude our message, wishing everyone a Happy Thanksgiving, I'm overcome with a sense of hope and renewed purpose. "If you're by yourself, don't be afraid to reach out to people because people do care, alright," I add, thinking of those who might be struggling, feeling alone. If my ordeal has taught me anything, it's the power of community, of reaching out, of allowing others to help.

We end the recording, and I pull Teri close, pressing a kiss to her forehead. "Happy Thanksgiving, baby," I murmur. As we stand there, in our home, surrounded by the scents and sounds of the holiday, I'm filled with an overwhelming sense of gratitude. For life, for health, for the incredible support system we have. This Thanksgiving isn't just a holiday – it's a celebration of survival, of love, of the indomitable human spirit. And as we prepare to sit down to our meal, I silently vow to carry this gratitude with me every day, to never again take for granted the simple joy of being alive and surrounded by love.

The journey continues with more dialysis training. I find myself back in the clinic, the familiar hum of machines a constant backdrop. Marta, my training nurse, stands beside me, her keen eyes watching my every move as I go through the process of setting up the dialysis machine.

"What's wrong? Good," I say, a hint of defensiveness in my voice as I fumble with a piece of equipment. Despite my progress, there's still so much to learn, so many ways to make mistakes. The weight of responsibility – this machine is literally keeping me alive – sometimes feels overwhelming.

Marta's voice cuts through my thoughts. "I tell you when there's something wrong, I will say hey! Hold on." Her tone is firm but not unkind. She's been patient throughout this process, but I know she needs to ensure I can do this correctly every single time.

As I continue setting up, Marta interjects again. "If I were you, I would not try to put that amount of tape." I resist the urge to sigh in frustration. Every step seems to come with a critique, a correction. But I remind myself that this is all part of the learning process, that Marta's attention to detail could very well save my life one day.

"Okay, that's fine," Marta says after a moment, and I feel a small surge of pride. It's a minor victory, but in this new reality where my life revolves around dialysis and medical procedures, I'll take whatever wins I can get.

As we continue the training session, I find myself reflecting on how far I've come. Just weeks ago, the idea of managing my own dialysis seemed impossibly daunting. Now, while still challenging, it's becoming more familiar, more manageable. Each session, each correction from Marta, brings me one step closer to independence, to regaining control over my life and health.

The training is grueling, both physically and mentally. By the end of each session, I'm exhausted, my mind swimming with procedures and precautions. But there's also a sense of accomplishment, of progress. This knowledge, these skills I'm acquiring, they're my ticket to a more normal life. They're the tools that will allow me to travel, to work, to live without being tethered to a hospital.

As I finish the setup and Marta gives her final approval for the day, I feel a mix of relief and determination. This is my new reality, and while it's not what I would have chosen, I'm determined to master it. Because beyond the tubes and machines and medical jargon lies the promise of life – of more days with my family, more opportunities to pursue my passions, more chances to make a difference in the world.

I pack up my things, thanking Marta for her patience and expertise. As I leave the clinic, I take a deep breath of the fresh outside air. Another day, another step forward. The journey is far from over, but with each passing day, I'm growing stronger, more confident, more hopeful about the future that lies ahead.

December 18th arrives with a crisp chill in the air, a stark contrast to the warmth of anticipation I feel as I pull into the parking garage of the Ascension Seton Abdominal Transplant clinic. This day marks a significant milestone in my journey – the restart of my kidney transplant referral process.

As I sit in my car, gathering my thoughts before heading in, I feel compelled to document this moment. I pull out my phone, the act of recording having become second nature over the past weeks.

"Today is December 18th. It's a Monday," I begin, my voice steady despite the nervous energy thrumming through me. "I am here at the Ascension Seton Abdominal Transplant clinic. I'm restarting the process for a kidney transplant referral, and I'm being evaluated today."

The weight of those words hits me as I speak them. This evaluation could be the first step towards a new kidney, towards freedom from dialysis, towards a return to normalcy. It's a hope I've been carrying for months, a light at the end of this long, challenging tunnel.

I make my way into the clinic, the sterile smell of disinfectant hitting me as I push through the doors. It's a scent I've become all too familiar with, but today it carries a note of hope. I'm directed to an evaluation room, where I settle in to wait, my mind racing with questions and possibilities.

As I sit there, surrounded by medical posters and the soft hum of equipment, I find myself reflecting on the journey that's brought me to this point. "One thing that was a surprise to me," I say to my phone camera, needing to vocalize my thoughts, "I started this process back in January, February of last year, continued until about May, and then lost communication with them. But what I learned today was one of the steps that I had taken... I thought that there were two things that were keeping me from moving forward."

I pause, gathering my thoughts. The complexity of this process never ceases to amaze me. "One was a colonoscopy, which I actually just had about a month ago in the hospital, and I gave them the report for that. And the other one was a cardiac clearance test."

As I speak, I'm struck by how much has changed since I first started this process. The urgency of my recent hospitalization, the grueling dialysis treatments, the overwhelming support from friends and family – all of it has shaped my perspective, making this moment feel all the more significant.

"I remember doing a cardiac clearance test, but I figured they needed to do another one or just needed to do one. I thought it was inconclusive, but what actually happened was I failed the previous one, for lack of a better term."

The realization sends a chill through me. It's a stark reminder of the complexities of my medical history, of the long-lasting impacts of my first bout with kidney failure. "Apparently, there was some kind of indication of a previous stent or a blockage, and that goes back to 2009 when I first got sick with my first kidney failure diagnosis."

Memories of that time flood back – the fear, the uncertainty, the physical toll of my body retaining so much fluid. "I got up to about 300 lbs. of fluid in addition to my body weight, and I had a heart event. I had a very brief stay in a hospital where they did a stent, and apparently that showed up on the cardiac clearance test."

As I recount this history, I'm struck by the resilience of the human body, and of the human spirit. I've been through so much, and yet here I am, still fighting, still hoping for a better future.

"But the strange thing is that it didn't stop me from being transplanted the first time," I muse, a note of confusion in my voice. "I'm not sure if this team is doing a more thorough job."

The uncertainty of it all weighs on me. Will this cardiac issue delay my chances for a transplant? Are there other hurdles I'm not yet aware of? But even as these questions swirl in my mind, I feel a sense of determination. I've come too far to give up now. Whatever challenges lie ahead, I'll face them head-on, just as I've faced every other obstacle in this journey.

A knock at the door interrupts my thoughts. It's time for the evaluation to begin. I take a deep breath, steeling myself for whatever comes next. This is just another step in the process, I remind myself. Another hurdle to clear on the path to healing, to reclaiming my life. With one last glance at the camera, I end the recording and prepare to meet with the transplant team.

Weeks pass, a blur of dialysis treatments, doctor's appointments, and small victories. And then, almost before I know it, I find myself back in a hospital room, this time for a procedure I've been both anticipating and dreading: the removal of my hemodialysis port.

As I lie on the hospital bed, the familiar beep of monitors in the background, I feel a mix of emotions. This port has been a constant companion since my hospitalization, a visible reminder of how close I came to the edge. It saved my life, facilitating the treatments that pulled me back from the brink. And now, it's time to say goodbye.

I reach for my phone, compelled as always to document this moment. "I'm getting my hemodialysis port removed today," I explain to the camera, my voice a mix of nervousness and excitement. "This is what saved my life in the hospital and helped me lose about 30 lbs. in a week. But it'll be coming out now. I'll be able to shower a lot easier."

As I speak, I run my fingers over the port, feeling its contours beneath my skin. It's strange to think of how quickly I've become accustomed to its presence, how it's become a part of me. Its removal feels symbolic – a step towards normalcy, towards health, towards a future less defined by my illness.

The medical team arrives, and I set my phone aside, taking deep breaths to calm my nerves. The procedure itself is a blur of sensations – the cool antiseptic on my skin, the pinch of the local anesthetic, the strange tugging feeling as they work to remove the port. I focus on my breathing, on the promise of what this removal means.

Before I know it, it's over. I pick up my phone again, eager to share the experience. "Well, they just took it out," I say, my voice a bit shaky. "That was stressful. The pain shots were ironically painful. But it was a very quick procedure, I don't know for sure."

As I speak, I gingerly touch the bandage where the port used to be. There's discomfort, yes, but also a sense of lightness. One less tube, one less tether to the medical equipment that's dominated my life for so long.

Lying there, port-free for the first time in weeks, I'm overwhelmed by the symbolism of this moment. The removal of the port marks the end of one chapter and the beginning of another. It's a step towards reclaiming my body, my independence, my life.

I think back on the journey that's brought me to this point – the fear and pain of my initial hospitalization, the grueling dialysis treatments, the outpouring of support from loved ones, the small victories and setbacks along the way. Each step, each challenge, has led to this moment.

As the nurse comes in to check on me, I'm already thinking ahead. To showers without having to worry about the port, to shirts that won't bulge oddly, to a body that's one step closer to being fully my own again. There's still a long road ahead – more dialysis, the continued quest for a transplant, the ongoing management of my health. But this moment feels like a turning point.

I end the recording and let my phone rest on my chest, closing my eyes for a moment. The steady beep of the heart monitor, once a source of anxiety, now sounds almost triumphant. Each beep is a reminder – I'm here, I'm alive, I'm healing.

The journey is far from over. There are still challenges ahead, more hurdles to overcome. But as I lie here, one medical device lighter, I feel a renewed sense of hope and determination. Whatever comes next, I know I'm ready to face it. One day at a time, one step at a time, I'm reclaiming my life, my health, my future. And for now, that's more than enough.

Chapter 11: Hurdles and Hope (Part 1 Revised)

The cool air hits my face as I step out of the cardiologist's office, a whirlwind of emotions and information swirling in my mind. I reach for my phone, the act of recording now a reflexive comfort, a way to process the flood of medical jargon and implications I've just been presented with.

"I'm coming back from my cardiologist visit," I begin, my voice steadier than I feel. "My transplant team referred me. The issue is that I had an abnormal cardiac clearance test, and thankfully they explained a lot better to me what is going on with that."

As I speak, I can feel some of the tension that's been knotting my shoulders for weeks starting to ease. Understanding, even of difficult news, is infinitely preferable to the fear of the unknown that's been dogging me.

"I was under the impression that there was some sort of ticking time bomb going on with my heart. It's actually not the case." The relief in my voice is palpable. "The cardiac clearance test really measures temperature around different areas in the heart. There are parts of your heart that, once it's under duress, are supposed to warm up. Well, there's one specific area in my heart that did not warm up on the clearance test I took back in February or March last year. That was because of the past stent that I've had."

As I delve into the explanation, memories of my first battle with kidney failure in 2009 surface. The fear, the uncertainty, the physical toll of my body retaining so much fluid - it all comes rushing back. Suddenly, I'm no longer in the parking lot of the cardiologist's office in 2024. Instead, I'm thrust back to one of the worst days of my life - June 12, 2009.

The fluorescent lights of the South Austin Walmart buzz overhead as I shuffle my swollen, 300-pound frame through the aisles. It's early morning, and I'm killing time until the pharmacy opens. The prednisone prescription in my pocket represents hope - hope that I can control this sudden, terrifying weight gain that has bloated my once-athletic body.

Just a month ago, I had been 215 pounds, closing out a successful year of acting with "The Grapes of Wrath." Now, diagnosed with IgA nephropathy and without health insurance, I'm drowning in medical debt and my own body fluids.

As 9:00 AM approaches, I make my way to the pharmacy counter, acutely aware of how visible my invisible illness has made me. The irritation I feel towards the pharmacy tech is irrational, I know, but I can't shake it. And then...

The tightness in my back and left shoulder. The crushing weight on my chest, as if an elephant has decided to take a seat. The creeping realization: Is this a heart attack? At 34?

The rest is a blur - the 911 call, the ambulance ride, the emergency room. "Heart event due to rapid weight gain and fluid overload," they said. A stent placed through my groin.

I blink, and I'm back in the present, the memory fading but its implications echoing loudly in my mind. "The stent was a result of fluid overload that I had back in 2009 when I was first sick and gained a lot of weight for my first kidney failure and had a heart event," I explain into the phone, my voice shaky with the weight of the recollection.

I pause, letting the weight of those words sink in. It's strange to think about how much my body has been through, how many battles it's fought. "But I wouldn't consider myself a cardiac patient," I add, almost as much to reassure myself as to inform anyone listening.

The good news, the doctor's reassuring words, tumble out next. "But the good news is the doctor told me that it's something that is very possibly reversible. It's not long-term damage, but their main concern is not that this would disqualify me from transplantation, but that I do have some kind of history of a heart event or some kind of heart attack and there's some narrowing of some blood vessels."

Hope mingles with caution in my voice as I continue. "But they said despite that evidence, I am in great shape. I exercise a lot, but the main concern is that they don't want there to be an actual heart attack during a transplant operation. They want to avoid that altogether."

I outline the next steps - retrieving old records, possibly another stent, maybe some aspirin therapy. It's a lot to process, but I feel a sense of forward momentum. "Everything's moving in the right direction. It's just another hurdle, but I feel pretty good about where we are now."

As I end the recording and slide into my car, I take a deep breath. This journey has been full of unexpected twists and turns, each new piece of information reshaping my understanding of my own body and health. But with each hurdle cleared, each question answered, I feel myself getting closer to the ultimate goal - a successful transplant and a return to health.

I start the car, ready to head home and share this news with Teri. There's still a long road ahead, but for the first time in a while, I feel like I can see where it's leading. And more importantly, I understand how my past is shaping my present and future. It's a sobering realization, but also an empowering one. Armed with this knowledge, I feel more prepared than ever to face whatever challenges lie ahead.

[The rest of Part 1 continues as before...]

Chapter 11: Hurdles and Hope (Part 1)

The cool air hits my face as I step out of the cardiologist's office, a whirlwind of emotions and information swirling in my mind. I reach for my phone, the act of recording now a reflexive comfort, a way to process the flood of medical jargon and implications I've just been presented with.

"I'm coming back from my cardiologist visit," I begin, my voice steadier than I feel. "My transplant team referred me. The issue is that I had an abnormal cardiac clearance test, and thankfully they explained a lot better to me what is going on with that."

As I speak, I can feel some of the tension that's been knotting my shoulders for weeks starting to ease. Understanding, even of difficult news, is infinitely preferable to the fear of the unknown that's been dogging me.

"I was under the impression that there was some sort of ticking time bomb going on with my heart. It's actually not the case." The relief in my voice is palpable. "The cardiac clearance test really measures temperature around different areas in the heart. There are parts of your heart that, once it's under duress, are supposed to warm up. Well, there's one specific area in my heart that did not warm up on the clearance test I took back in February or March last year. That was because of the past stent that I've had."

As I delve into the explanation, memories of my first battle with kidney failure in 2009 surface. The fear, the uncertainty, the physical toll of my body retaining so much fluid - it all comes rushing back. "The stent was a result of fluid overload that I had back in 2009 when I was first sick and gained a lot of weight for my first kidney failure and had a heart event."

I pause, letting the weight of those words sink in. It's strange to think about how much my body has been through, how many battles it's fought. "But I wouldn't consider myself a cardiac patient," I add, almost as much to reassure myself as to inform anyone listening.

The good news, the doctor's reassuring words, tumble out next. "But the good news is the doctor told me that it's something that is very possibly reversible. It's not long-term damage, but their main concern is not that this would disqualify me from transplantation, but that I do have some kind of history of a heart event or some kind of heart attack and there's some narrowing of some blood vessels."

Hope mingles with caution in my voice as I continue. "But they said despite that evidence, I am in great shape. I exercise a lot, but the main concern is that they don't want there to be an actual heart attack during a transplant operation. They want to avoid that altogether."

I outline the next steps - retrieving old records, possibly another stent, maybe some aspirin therapy. It's a lot to process, but I feel a sense of forward momentum. "Everything's moving in the right direction. It's just another hurdle, but I feel pretty good about where we are now."

As I end the recording and slide into my car, I take a deep breath. This journey has been full of unexpected twists and turns, each new piece of information reshaping my understanding of my own body and health. But with each hurdle cleared, each question answered, I feel myself getting closer to the ultimate goal - a successful transplant and a return to health.

I start the car, ready to head home and share this news with Teri. There's still a long road ahead, but for the first time in a while, I feel like I can see where it's leading.

The scenery blurs past as I drive home from my gastroenterology follow-up, my mind racing even faster than the car. I feel compelled to record my thoughts, to make sense of this latest development in my ongoing medical saga.

"Now I'm riding home," I begin, my voice a mix of weariness and determination. "I just had a gastroenterology follow-up from my stay in the hospital. I was told by my Cardiology team that I actually needed to have a gastroenterology follow-up to rule out any potential bleeding that I might be having."

As I speak, I'm struck by the interconnectedness of it all - how one medical issue leads to another, how each specialist's findings ripple out to affect my overall treatment plan. It's a complex dance, and I'm still learning the steps.

"We never really did find any the first time when I went to the hospital, but they thought that it might be gastritis," I continue, recalling the uncertainty of those early days in the hospital. The memory of that time - the fear, the pain, the not knowing - still has the power to make my heart race.

"My specialist doesn't really feel that I am in danger of losing any blood right now, but we went ahead and scheduled me for a pill cam," I explain, a note of curiosity creeping into my voice. The idea of swallowing a tiny camera, of it traveling through my body and documenting my insides, feels like something out of a science fiction movie.

"Now I'll swallow a pill. It will take pictures of my insides for about eight hours and then I'll turn the data in and they'll see if there's any bleeding from my small intestine which they couldn't get with the colonoscopy or the endoscopy."

As I finish recording and focus back on the road, I'm struck by the strange journey my body has become. From dialysis to heart tests to swallowable cameras - it's a far cry from the life I was living just months ago. But each test, each procedure, is a step towards answers, towards health, towards a future where my body is my own again.

I pull into my driveway, ready to share this latest development with Teri. Tomorrow will bring new challenges, new questions. But for now, I allow myself to feel a glimmer of hope. We're moving forward, one test at a time.

The soft glow of my computer screen illuminates my home office as I settle in to record the latest update in my ongoing medical journey. The familiar weight of my phone in my hand is comforting as I begin to speak.

"I got a call from the transplant coordinator," I start, my voice a mix of anticipation and apprehension. "They let me know that they did put my case before the board on January 10th. That was a Wednesday."

I pause, remembering the flutter of nerves I felt when I saw the coordinator's number pop up on my phone. Every call, every piece of communication feels loaded with potential - the potential for good news, for progress, or for yet another setback.

"They marked my file as incomplete," I continue, a hint of frustration creeping into my tone. "Because they're still waiting to find out about the Cardiology report and the heart cath, which will hopefully be resolved in February with another follow-up in March to see how I'm progressing."

As I speak, I'm acutely aware of the passage of time. Each day, each week that passes is another day of dialysis, another day of waiting, another day of my life on hold. The process feels endless sometimes, a constant cycle of tests and appointments and waiting for results.

"No positive answers yet," I admit, "but I'm moving in the right direction, which is better than being outright denied."

I end the recording and lean back in my chair, letting out a long breath. The weight of uncertainty settles on my shoulders like a familiar, if unwelcome, companion. It's a strange limbo to be in - not approved, but not denied. Moving forward, but at a pace that sometimes feels glacial.

As I sit there in the quiet of my office, I'm struck by the resilience this journey has demanded of me. Each hurdle cleared, each test endured, each piece of uncertain news weathered - it's all part of the process. A process that's reshaping not just my body, but my understanding of patience, of perseverance, of hope.

I glance at the calendar on my desk, my eyes automatically finding the dates of my upcoming appointments. February for the heart cath, March for the follow-up. Each date a potential turning point, a possible step closer to the transplant I so desperately need.

With a sigh, I push myself up from my chair. There's nothing to do now but wait, to continue with my dialysis, to take care of myself as best I can. And to hold onto hope - hope that each day brings me closer to health, to wholeness, to a life no longer defined by illness and uncertainty.

As I leave my office, switching off the light, I make a silent promise to myself. No matter how long this journey takes, no matter how many hurdles I have to clear, I won't give up. I'll keep moving forward, one day at a time, one test at a time, one small victory at a time. Because at the end of this long road, health and a new kidney await. And that's worth every struggle, every setback, every moment of uncertainty. That's worth fighting for.

Chapter 11: Hurdles and Hope (Part 2 Revised)

The harsh fluorescent lights of the hospital room cast a sickly glow over my skin as I settle onto the bed, the familiar beep of monitors a discordant lullaby. It's February 11th, a date that should be filled with celebration - my oldest son's 20th birthday. Instead, I find myself back in the hospital, a place that's become all too familiar over the past months.

I reach for my phone, the act of recording now a comforting ritual in times of stress and uncertainty. "Well, it looks like I'm back in the hospital," I begin, my voice tinged with a mix of resignation and frustration. "It is February 11th. It's actually my oldest son's 20th birthday. I was in the hospital 20 years ago for a different reason, but I'm here because last night I had a very immense pain when I started my dialysis treatment and I couldn't go past maybe about a minute."

As I speak, I can feel the echo of that pain, the searing agony that had me gasping for breath, unable to continue with the life-saving treatment my body so desperately needs. "I knew that doing this for an hour, let alone nine hours, was unsustainable," I continue, the memory making me wince.

The events of the past night replay in my mind, vivid and jarring. It had been a Friday night like any other, the dialysis machine humming in the background, a sound as familiar as my own heartbeat. I was settling in for my nightly treatment when that sharp pain lanced through my abdomen.

At first, I tried to brush it off. Pain wasn't uncommon in this journey, after all. But as the minutes ticked by, the pain intensified, transforming from a nuisance to a roaring, all-consuming agony.

"Teri," I had called out, my voice tight with pain. "Something's wrong."

What followed was a blur of phone calls and increasing discomfort. We dialed the overnight health line for the dialysis center, waiting on hold as the pain crescendoed. After what felt like an eternity, but was probably closer to 30 minutes, we finally got a call back.

The nurse on the other end of the line ran through a checklist of procedures. "Have you tried repositioning the catheter? Flushing the line?"

"Yes, yes," I replied, frustration mounting. "I've done all of that. Nothing's helping."

Now, as I recount the events to the camera, I can still feel the urgency of that midnight drive to the ER, see the fluorescent lights of the emergency room, the looks of concern from the night shift nurses. It was all cinematic in a way I wished it wasn't.

"It turns out I have peritonitis," I explain to the camera, the medical term feeling heavy on my tongue. "Which is an inflammation of the peritoneum when you get peritoneal dialysis. That's a danger that can happen if you get infected."

The word 'peritonitis' hangs in the air, another medical term to add to the ever-growing lexicon of my illness. Another complication, another setback in a journey that sometimes feels endless.

"They gave me some IVs and something for the pain, but hopefully I'll be out of here in a couple of days and back on track," I say, trying to inject a note of optimism into my voice. But even as I speak the words, I'm aware of the toll this latest setback is taking, not just physically, but emotionally.

The weekend passes in a haze of antibiotics and pain medication. I drift in and out of consciousness, aware on some level that this is a setback, another hurdle in my quest to get on the transplant list. In my more lucid moments, I worry about how this will affect my chances.

Monday morning arrives, and with it, a new challenge. Instead of the support I desperately need, I'm met with suspicion at the dialysis clinic.

"Mr. Pouhé," the nurse begins, her tone more accusatory than concerned, "peritonitis is often the result of improper cleaning techniques. Are you sure you've been following all the protocols?"

I feel a surge of indignation. "Of course I have," I reply, my voice hoarse from the weekend's ordeal. "I'm meticulous about my procedures."

But my protests seem to fall on deaf ears. "We'll need to schedule an early home inspection," she continues. "To rule out anything in your environment that might be causing this."

As I leave the clinic, I feel a weight of frustration and worry settling on my shoulders. This isn't just about the pain or the inconvenience. This is a threat to everything I've been working towards.

That night, as I set up for dialysis - a process now tinged with new anxiety - I turn to the camera once again. "So, here's a plot twist I didn't see coming," I begin, my voice betraying my exhaustion and frustration. "Peritonitis. It's like my body has turned against itself, and now the very people who are supposed to be helping me seem to think it's my fault."

I pause, collecting my thoughts. "You know, throughout this whole journey, I've tried to be the perfect patient. I've followed every rule, dotted every 'i', crossed every 't'. And now, to have them look at me with suspicion... it's hard. It's really hard."

Teri's voice comes from behind the camera, soft and supportive. "But you know you've done everything right."

I nod, feeling a lump form in my throat. "I have. But what if it doesn't matter? What if this setback, this... this betrayal by my own body, costs me my shot at the transplant list?"

As I connect myself to the dialysis machine, my movements now tinged with a new caution, I can't help but reflect on the precariousness of my situation. Every infection, every complication, feels like it could be the one to derail everything.

"This is the part of the story they don't tell you about," I say to the camera, my voice low. "The constant vigilance, the fear that despite your best efforts, something could go wrong. And when it does, you're not just fighting the illness. You're fighting the system, fighting to be believed, fighting to hold onto hope."

The dialysis machine beeps, signaling the start of another session. As the familiar process begins, I find myself staring at the catheter site, now a source of both life-saving treatment and potential danger.

"But here's the thing," I continue, a note of determination creeping into my voice. "This is just another chapter in the story. It's not the end. I'll get through this inspection, I'll prove that I've been doing everything right, and I'll keep pushing forward. Because that's what this journey is about. It's not just about the medical procedures or the waiting. It's about perseverance. It's about hope."

As I end the recording, I'm exhausted but resolute. This setback with peritonitis, the suspicion from the medical staff - it's not the end of my story. It's just another chapter, another hurdle to overcome. And overcome it I will, camera in hand, capturing every step of the way. Because this journey, with all its ups and downs, is a story that needs to be told. A story of resilience, of hope, and of the complex, often frustrating world of healthcare that so many navigate in silence.

[We're going to make a new pill cam chapter.]

Chapter 12: Under the Microscope

The day of the home inspection looms like a storm on the horizon. I've spent the days leading up to it in a frenzy of cleaning and organizing, even though I know my dialysis area is already meticulously maintained. It's not just about passing the inspection; it's about vindicating myself, proving that the peritonitis wasn't due to any negligence on my part.

As I set up the camera that morning, I can't keep the edge out of my voice. "Welcome to inspection day," I say, gesturing around our guest room-turned-dialysis-den. "Where we prove that yes, I do know how to keep things clean."

Teri places a calming hand on my shoulder. "They're just doing their job, Marc. Try to remember that."

I nod, taking a deep breath. She's right, of course. But it's hard not to feel like I'm on trial.

The doorbell rings at precisely 10 AM. Two nurses from the dialysis clinic, armed with clipboards and serious expressions, stand on our doorstep. I usher them in, fighting the urge to launch into a preemptive defense of my practices.

"Mr. Pouhé," the lead nurse begins, her tone professional but not unkind. "We'll need to see your dialysis area and go through your entire procedure. Please walk us through it as if you were starting your nightly treatment."

I nod, leading them to the guest room. As we enter, I can't help but feel a surge of pride. The room is spotless, every surface gleaming, supplies neatly organized. I've even labeled everything with a label maker, a touch of obsessive organization that I hope will impress.

"This is where the magic happens," I say, attempting to inject some levity into the situation. The nurses don't smile, but I press on. "Shall we begin?"

For the next two hours, I walk them through every step of my dialysis routine. I demonstrate my hand-washing technique, show them how I clean the catheter site, explain my system for keeping everything sterile. I feel like a performer on stage, hyper-aware of every movement, every word.

The nurses take copious notes, occasionally asking questions or requesting that I repeat a step. Their faces remain impassive, giving no hint as to what they're thinking.

As we near the end of the inspection, the lead nurse speaks up. "Mr. Pouhé, can you show us your supply storage area?"

I lead them to the closet where I keep my dialysis supplies. As I open the door, I hold my breath, praying that nothing will be out of place.

The nurse examines the shelves, checking expiration dates and storage conditions. After what feels like an eternity, she turns to me. "Your organization is... impressive," she says, a note of surprise in her voice.

I feel a weight lift from my shoulders. "Thank you," I reply, trying to keep the relief out of my voice. "I take this very seriously."

As the inspection concludes, the nurses huddle in our living room, speaking in low voices and making final notes on their clipboards. The wait is excruciating.

Finally, the lead nurse approaches me. "Mr. Pouhé, based on what we've seen today, we can confidently say that your home dialysis setup and procedures meet all of our standards. In fact, your attention to detail is exemplary."

The relief that washes over me is almost physical. "So, you don't think the peritonitis was caused by anything I did?"

She shakes her head. "Sometimes, despite our best efforts, infections can occur. Your practices are not to blame. We'll note in your file that your home care is excellent."

As the nurses leave, I feel a complex mix of emotions - relief, vindication, but also a lingering frustration that I'd had to prove myself in the first place.

That evening, as I set up for dialysis, I turn to the camera. "Well, we passed with flying colors," I say, a wry smile on my face. "Turns out I do know how to keep things clean. Who would have thought?"

Teri's voice comes from behind the camera. "How do you feel?"

I pause, considering. "Relieved, mostly. But also... I don't know. It's frustrating that I had to go through all this, that they assumed I must have done something wrong. It makes you feel... vulnerable. Like you're always one step away from being blamed for something beyond your control."

As I connect myself to the dialysis machine, I continue to reflect. "You know, this whole experience - the peritonitis, the accusation, this inspection - it's really highlighted something about this journey. It's not just about the physical challenges. It's about constantly having to advocate for yourself, to prove yourself. Even to the people who are supposed to be on your side."

I look directly into the camera. "I think that's an important part of this story. The emotional toll of always being under scrutiny, of feeling like you can't afford to make a single mistake. Because it's not just about your health - it's about your chances at a new life."

As the dialysis begins, I find myself thinking about how to incorporate this experience into the documentary. The tension of the inspection, the vindication of passing - it's all compelling stuff. But more than that, it's a window into the psychological challenges of living with a chronic illness, of being constantly at the mercy of a complex and sometimes skeptical medical system.

"Maybe that's the real story here," I muse aloud. "Not just the medical procedures or the wait for a transplant, but the human experience of it all. The fear, the frustration, the small victories. The way it changes how you see yourself and the world around you."

Teri steps out from behind the camera, sitting beside me. "I think you're onto something there," she says softly.

As the night wears on, my mind is already piecing together scenes, thinking about how to visually represent the feeling of being under constant scrutiny. The inspection has been a hurdle, yes, but it has also given me new insight into the story I'm trying to tell.

This journey isn't just about getting a new kidney. It's about maintaining your dignity, your sense of self, in the face of a system that often seems designed to strip those things away. It's about finding strength and resilience in unexpected places.

As I drift off to sleep, the dialysis machine humming its familiar lullaby, I feel a renewed sense of purpose. We've cleared another hurdle, yes. But more than that, we've uncovered another layer of this complex, challenging, but ultimately human story. And it's a story I'm more determined than ever to tell.

Chapter 13: A Journey Within

The morning of the pill cam procedure dawns bright and clear, a stark contrast to the anxiety churning in my gut. As I prepare to leave for the gastroenterology appointment, I find myself reaching for the camera, a now-familiar gesture of documentation and self-reflection.

"Yes, cool. I'm driving to my gastroenterology appointment," I begin, my voice a mix of nervousness and curiosity. "I'm about to swallow a pill cam. It's going to take pictures of my insides to identify the source of any bleeding if there is any. That's what we suspected when I got several bags of blood transfusions back in November."

As I speak, the reality of what I'm about to do hits me. A tiny camera, traveling through my body, capturing images of my insides. It's like something out of a science fiction movie, yet here I am, about to experience it firsthand.

The drive to the hospital is a blur of thoughts and worries. What if they find something serious? What if they don't find anything at all, leaving us back at square one? And perhaps most pressingly, what if I can't swallow the pill? It's not exactly a normal-sized capsule, after all.

In the waiting room, I fidget with the hem of my shirt, my mind racing. When the nurse calls my name, I stand on slightly shaky legs. This is it.

The procedure itself is surprisingly anticlimactic. The pill cam, while larger than your average medication, goes down easily with a glass of water. As I swallow, I can't help but think about the journey it's about to embark on, the hidden landscapes of my own body it will reveal.

"Alright, Mr. Pouhé," the nurse says, helping me into a harness-like contraption. "This belt will pick up the signals from the pill cam. You'll need to wear it for the next eight hours."

As I leave the hospital, I feel like a walking science experiment. The belt around my abdomen, the wires snaking up to a small receiver - it's all a very visible reminder of the invisible process happening inside me.

Back in the car, I turn the camera on again, feeling the need to document this strange experience. "I'm heading home now," I say, panning down to show the equipment. "You can see everything I'm wearing. I had to wear this belt around my abdomen. The cables wrap around me."

I hold up the receiver, its blinking blue light a constant reminder of the tiny explorer making its way through my body. "I don't know if you can see that, but that's the flashing blue light for the receiver. It's picking up signals from the pill cam as it travels through my intestinal tract."

As I drive home, I'm acutely aware of every bump in the road, every turn. Is it affecting the camera's journey? Will it impact the images? It's strange to think that right now, at this very moment, a part of me that I've never seen and will never see with my own eyes is being photographed, documented, studied.

The day passes slowly. I try to go about my normal routine, but it's hard to forget about the camera inside me. Every twinge, every gurgle takes on new significance. Is that the pill cam making its way through? Did it just capture an image of something important?

In the quiet moments, my mind wanders to the bigger picture. "This is another hurdle for my upcoming transplant evaluation," I muse aloud to the camera. "Hopefully between this and my heart cath, which has been pushed back once already to March 5th and the follow-up for that in April, I can be on the transplant list by late April to early May."

I allow myself a moment of hope, picturing a future where these hurdles are behind me, where a new kidney and a new lease on life await. "Hopefully, I will be transplanted sometime this summer," I say, the words carrying the weight of all my hopes and fears.

But even as I voice this optimism, I can feel the toll this journey is taking. "I really hope all these extra steps have worked," I admit, a note of vulnerability creeping into my voice, "because I am really tired."

As evening approaches, it's time to return to the hospital to have the equipment removed and the data collected. In the car, I find myself talking to the camera again, processing the day's events.

"I'm back a few minutes early to get my pill-cam data evaluated," I explain. "They're about to go and pull the data from it now. My gastroenterologist is going to evaluate it. They said it could take two to three weeks to know the results."

As I hand over the equipment, I feel a mix of relief and anticipation. The physical process is over, but now comes the waiting. More waiting, always waiting.

"Here's hoping everything is clear," I say to the camera as I leave the hospital. "Or here's hoping that there's an easily identifiable problem that we can fix."

Driving home, I reflect on the uniqueness of this experience. For one day, I've had a window into the inner workings of my own body. It's both fascinating and humbling, a reminder of the complex, intricate processes happening inside us every moment of every day.

But more than that, it's a reminder of the journey I'm on. A journey not just through the medical system, not just towards a hopeful transplant, but a journey of self-discovery. With each test, each procedure, I'm learning more about my body, about my resilience, about the limits of my patience and the depths of my determination.

As I pull into my driveway, I take a moment to sit in the stillness of the car. The pill cam has completed its journey, but mine continues. There will be more tests, more waiting, more hurdles to clear. But for now, I allow myself to feel a small sense of accomplishment. One more step taken, one more piece of the puzzle in place.

I reach for the camera one last time. "Whatever the results," I say, looking directly into the lens, "we keep moving forward. That's what this whole journey is about. Forward motion, no matter what."

With that, I turn off the camera and head inside. Tomorrow will bring new challenges, new worries. But tonight, I've traveled a journey within myself, both literally and figuratively. And somehow, that makes me feel more prepared for whatever comes next.

Chapter 14: The Waiting Game

The months following my evaluation blend into a surreal routine of medical appointments and administrative battles. Each day brings a new challenge, a delicate balance between nurturing hope for a transplant and navigating the labyrinth of healthcare bureaucracy.

My evenings, once a time for relaxation, have become dedicated to what I've begun to think of as my "second job" - battling the healthcare system. Hours are spent on hold, navigating automated phone systems, and arguing with various representatives.

Today, I find myself once again on the phone, this time with Sarah, the Abdominal Transplant Center's financial coordinator. The $2,300 bill from the third-party lab facility looms large in my mind as I explain the situation for what feels like the hundredth time.

"I understand your frustration, Mr. Pouhé," Sarah says, her voice a mix of sympathy and professional detachment. "But without the proper documentation from the transplant team, my hands are tied."

I take a deep breath, trying to keep my composure. "But the transplant team sent me to that lab," I explain, for what must be the dozenth time. "How can they not be responsible for ensuring the proper paperwork was filed?"

"I hear you," Sarah replies, "but the issue is that we don't have any record of the orders for those tests. Without that, we can't authorize payment or submit it to your insurance."

It's a maddening cycle, one I've been trapped in for weeks. I thank Sarah for her time, knowing full well that this conversation, like so many before it, has led nowhere.

Determined to make some progress, I decide to try contacting the third-party lab directly. After navigating another labyrinthine phone system, I finally reach a billing specialist.

"I'm sorry, sir," the specialist tells me after I explain my situation, "but we can only bill based on the orders we receive. If we don't have proper documentation from the ordering physician, we have to bill you directly."

I feel my frustration mounting. "But I didn't just walk in off the street," I argue. "I was sent there by my transplant team. Surely there must be some record of that?"

"I understand, but without the actual orders, there's nothing we can do on our end," comes the reply.

As I hang up the phone, a realization begins to dawn on me. I've been approaching this from the wrong angle. What I need is to get all these parties communicating with each other, with the transplant doctor at the center.

With renewed determination, I dial the transplant center again, this time asking specifically to leave a message for my transplant doctor.

"Dr. Johnson," I say into the voicemail, "I'm sorry to bother you with this, but I'm at my wit's end. There's a $2,300 bill from the lab you sent me to that's been in dispute for months. The financial coordinator can't help without your orders, and the lab says the same thing. Is there any way you can reach out to both of them and clarify that these tests were ordered by you? I'm worried this could affect my chances of being listed for transplant."

As I end the message, I feel a mix of hope and anxiety. Will this finally be the key to resolving this issue? Or am I just adding another layer to an already complex situation?

The next day, as I'm setting up for my nightly dialysis, my phone rings. It's Dr. Johnson's office.

"Mr. Pouhé," the nurse says, "Dr. Johnson asked me to call you. He's reviewed your file and reached out to both the lab and our financial department. He's confirmed that the tests were ordered by our team and has sent the necessary documentation to both parties."

I feel a wave of relief wash over me. "So does this mean the bill will be taken care of?"

"It should be," the nurse replies. "Dr. Johnson has asked the financial department to process it as soon as possible and submit it to your insurance. You should be receiving an updated statement soon."

As I hang up the phone, I'm struck by a mix of emotions. Relief, certainly, that this particular battle seems to be nearing its end. But also frustration that it took so much time and effort to resolve what should have been a simple administrative task.

I turn to the camera, feeling the need to document this moment. "You know," I begin, "I never thought I'd feel this excited about paperwork. But this... this feels like a victory. A small one, maybe, in the grand scheme of things. But when you're in this situation, fighting for your health on one front and fighting the system on another, every win counts."

I pause, considering the broader implications of what I've just been through. "It shouldn't be this hard," I continue. "Patients shouldn't have to become expert negotiators and administrators just to get the care they need. But here we are. And if sharing this story can help even one person navigate this maze a little more easily, then maybe all this frustration will have been worth it."

As I start my dialysis for the night, I find myself feeling cautiously optimistic. This billing issue, which has been hanging over my head for months, seems to be resolving. It's a reminder that persistence pays off, that it's worth fighting for what you need.

But it's also a stark reminder of the complexities of the healthcare system, of the many obstacles that stand between patients and the care they need. As I drift off to sleep, the dialysis machine humming softly in the background, I can't help but wonder: how many others are out there, fighting these same battles? And what can be done to make the system work better for those it's meant to serve?

The waiting game continues. But tonight, at least, I feel like I've taken a step forward. And in this journey, every step counts.

Chapter 15: A Beacon of Hope

Dr. Lappin's words hang in the air, each one carrying the weight of possibility. "We've been contacted by someone who wants to be a living donor for you," she continues, her voice steady but tinged with excitement. "They've volunteered to participate in the donor exchange program on your behalf."

The revelation hits me like a physical force, a jolt of electricity that courses through my body. In all the chaos of the past months - the endless medical appointments, the battles with insurance companies, the roller coaster of hope and despair - I had somehow pushed to the back of my mind this beacon of hope, this incredible act of selflessness.

As Dr. Lappin's words sink in, I find myself transported back to that Sunday in November, when I was first hospitalized. The memory washes over me, vivid and intense:

The fluorescent lights of the emergency room cast a harsh glow over everything, making the world feel surreal and slightly off-kilter. The beeping of monitors, the hushed voices of medical staff, the palpable tension in the air - it all blends into a cacophony of fear and uncertainty.

I'm lying on a gurney, my body swollen and aching, each breath a struggle. The weight of my illness, both physical and emotional, threatens to crush me. It's in this moment of darkness that a nurse approaches, a small smile on her face.

"Mr. Pouhé," she says, her voice a soothing counterpoint to the chaos around us, "someone's here to see you. A friend, I believe."

And there they are, stepping into view. Their name and face blur in my memory - whether from the fog of illness or the desire to protect their privacy, I'm not sure. But their presence, their words, are crystal clear.

"I want to help," they say, their voice filled with determination. "I want to be tested as a donor for you."

In that moment, amidst the fear and pain, a small flame of hope ignites in my chest.

The memory fades, and I'm back in Dr. Lappin's office, still reeling from her announcement.

"They've already begun their evaluation process," Dr. Lappin adds, pulling me back to the present. "They've been keeping you updated privately, haven't they?"

I nod, a lump forming in my throat. "Yes, they've been sending me texts and private messages on social media. They've been... incredibly kind."

A complex mix of emotions washes over me. Gratitude, certainly, for this person's incredible generosity. Hope, at the possibility of a faster path to transplant. But also, surprisingly, a twinge of discomfort.

Dr. Lappin must notice my conflicted expression. "I sense that their updates make you uncomfortable?" she probes gently.

I nod, struggling to articulate the tangle of feelings. "I'm incredibly grateful," I begin, "more than I can express. But my own journey has been so... complicated. There have been so many setbacks, so many hurdles. The thought of sharing all of that with them, of potentially disappointing them if something goes wrong..."

"That's a very normal way to feel," Dr. Lappin reassures me. "The transplant process is deeply personal, and everyone handles it differently. You're not obligated to share any more than you're comfortable with."

As I leave the transplant center that day, my mind is a whirlwind of thoughts and emotions. The elation of being listed for transplant is tempered by the weight of this new development. The potential donor's generosity is a gift beyond measure, but it also brings with it a new set of complex emotions to navigate.

Over the next few weeks, as I settle into the reality of being on the transplant list, I find myself grappling with how to handle the situation with my potential donor. Their private messages are filled with updates on their evaluation process, each one a mix of excitement and nerves.

"Just finished another round of tests! Fingers crossed everything looks good."

"Meeting with the transplant team next week. One step closer to helping you get a second chance at life!"

Each message fills me with a mixture of gratitude and anxiety. Their enthusiasm is touching, their commitment humbling. But with each update they share, I feel an increasing pressure to reciprocate, to open up about my own journey.

Yet something holds me back. The memory of all the setbacks, the billing disputes, the moments of despair - they feel too raw, too personal to share, even with someone who is offering me such an incredible gift. I fear that exposing the full complexity of my journey might somehow jinx this newfound hope, or worse, burden the very person who is already giving so much.

One evening, as I set up for my nightly dialysis, I find myself turning to the camera, needing to process these conflicting emotions.

"You know," I begin, my voice low and thoughtful, "I've been thinking a lot about names lately. About privacy and how much of ourselves we share with the world."

I pause, collecting my thoughts. "In telling this story, I've changed some names, especially of healthcare professionals and anyone directly involved in my care. It's not about hiding anything, but about protecting privacy, about recognizing that this journey affects more than just me."

I glance down at my phone, where the latest message from my potential donor glows on the screen. "And then there's this incredible person, this potential donor. They've revealed their name to my local community, but I don't feel comfortable sharing it this early in the story. It feels... premature, somehow. Like I'm getting ahead of myself."

I take a deep breath, feeling the weight of everything that's happened, everything that's still to come. "This journey... it's so personal, so intense. And now there's this other person, this beacon of hope, who's willing to go through so much for me. It's overwhelming, in the best and scariest ways possible."

As I connect myself to the dialysis machine, I find myself reflecting on the strange, beautiful complexity of human connection. Here I am, tethered to a machine that keeps me alive, while somewhere out there, a person I barely know is undergoing tests and evaluations, all in the hope of giving me a second chance at life.

The enormity of it all washes over me. The generosity of my potential donor, the skill and dedication of my medical team, the love and support of my family and friends - it's a tapestry of human kindness and resilience that leaves me humbled and grateful.

Yet even as I bask in this warmth, I'm acutely aware of the challenges that lie ahead. The road to transplant is long and uncertain, filled with potential pitfalls and setbacks. As much as I want to share every step of this journey with my potential donor, to let them know how much their gift means to me, I find myself holding back, protecting both of us from the weight of expectation.

As the dialysis machine hums softly in the background, I make a silent promise to myself. I will find a way to navigate this complex emotional landscape. I will honor the gift my potential donor is offering, while also honoring my own need for privacy and emotional space. And through it all, I will continue to document this journey, in all its messy, beautiful complexity.

Because at its heart, this isn't just my story. It's a story of human connection, of hope in the face of adversity, of the incredible things we can achieve when we come together. And that's a story worth telling, in all its intricate, nuanced glory.

Chapter 16: The Heart of the Matter

The incessant beeping of my alarm pierces the pre-dawn darkness, jolting me from a fitful sleep. It's 5:30 AM, and I'm already exhausted. Nine hours of dialysis the night before have left me drained, but there's no time to dwell on that now. Today is the day of my long-awaited, much-rescheduled heart catheterization.

As I slowly sit up, careful not to disturb the still-healing catheter site on my abdomen, memories of the past few weeks flood my mind. The constant back-and-forth with the cardiologist's office plays like a frustrating movie reel:

"Mr. Pouhé, I'm sorry, but we need to reschedule your heart catheterization again."

"But this is the third time you've changed the date. I need this for my transplant evaluation."

"I understand, sir, but we've had some scheduling conflicts. How about next Wednesday?"

Only to be followed by another call: "I'm sorry, Mr. Pouhé, but that Wednesday slot is no longer available. We'll have to push it to March."

Each conversation blends into the next, a blur of apologies, rescheduling, and growing frustration. February slipped away, and suddenly it was March, and I was still waiting.

The crescendo of this symphony of bureaucratic chaos came just yesterday, with an unexpected call from the transplant coordinator:

"Mr. Pouhé, I wanted to let you know as a courtesy that we had to present your case to the board. I'm afraid it was denied pending the heart catheterization results."

I remember how the air left my lungs at those words. "But I've been trying to get that scheduled for weeks!"

"I understand, and we did receive good results from your pill cam. But we need those heart cath results before we can move forward."

Now, as I carefully make my way to the bathroom to get ready, the weight of today's importance settles heavily on my shoulders. This isn't just another medical procedure. This is the key to unlocking my future, to moving forward with the transplant evaluation. Without it, I'm stuck in limbo, my health deteriorating while I wait for the medical bureaucracy to align.

Teri stirs as I exit the bathroom. "You ready?" she asks, her voice still thick with sleep.

I nod, not trusting my voice just yet. The truth is, I'm far from ready. I'm exhausted, frustrated, and more than a little scared. But I'm also determined. After months of delays and rescheduling, I'm not leaving that hospital without getting this procedure done.

The drive to the hospital is quiet, the pre-dawn streets nearly empty. As Teri navigates through the city, I find myself rehearsing what I'll say if they try to reschedule again. The polite, patient Marc is taking a backseat today. If necessary, I'm prepared to fight for my place in line.

We pull up to the valet stand, and as I hand over the keys, a sense of déjà vu washes over me. "We've been here before, haven't we?" I ask Teri as we walk towards the entrance.

She nods, a small smile on her face despite the early hour. "Last year, remember? For that consultation."

The memory clicks into place, adding another layer of surreality to the morning. How much has changed in a year, how much is still uncertain.

As we approach the check-in desk, I feel my anxiety rising. The receptionist looks up as we approach, her expression neutral. "Name, please?"

"Marc Pouhé," I respond, unable to keep the edge out of my voice. "I'm here for a heart catheterization."

She types something into her computer, then frowns slightly. My heart sinks. I know that look.

"I'm sorry, Mr. Pouhé, but it looks like your procedure has been pushed back. We had some emergency cases come in this morning."

And just like that, something snaps inside me. All the frustration, all the delays, all the conflicting information - it all comes boiling to the surface.

"Pushed back?" I repeat, my voice rising. I'm aware that I'm making a scene, but months of pent-up frustration are pouring out, and I can't seem to stop it. "I've been trying to get this procedure done for months. Months! Do you have any idea what this means for my transplant evaluation?"

The receptionist looks taken aback by my outburst. "Sir, I understand you're frustrated, but-"

"No, I don't think you do understand," I cut her off. "Every delay, every rescheduling, every mix-up - it's not just an inconvenience. It's my life on hold. It's my chance at a transplant slipping away."

Teri places a hand on my arm, a gentle reminder to calm down. But I'm too far gone. I need answers, and I need them now.

"I need to speak to someone in charge," I demand, my voice carrying across the now-silent waiting room.

As a harried-looking nurse hurries over to deal with the situation, I take a deep breath, trying to center myself. I know I'm walking a fine line here. I need to be forceful enough to be taken seriously, but not so aggressive that they refuse to help me.

"Look," I say, my voice lower but still intense, "I understand that emergencies happen. But I've been rescheduled multiple times. I'm in the middle of a transplant evaluation. Every delay puts my health at risk. There has to be something you can do."

The nurse, to her credit, listens patiently. When I finish, she nods. "Let me see what I can find out. Please, have a seat, and I'll be right back."

As Teri and I settle into the uncomfortable waiting room chairs, I feel a mix of emotions washing over me. Anger at the constant delays, fear about what this means for my transplant chances, guilt over causing a scene, and underneath it all, a bone-deep exhaustion.

"I'm sorry," I murmur to Teri. "I know I shouldn't have lost my temper like that."

She squeezes my hand. "Sometimes you have to advocate for yourself," she says softly. "You've been more than patient."

Her words remind me of something I've learned throughout this journey. Sometimes, you have to get mad. You have to be clear with your language, fierce in your determination. Especially when you look and sound like me - a middle-aged Black man in a medical system that doesn't always listen to people who look like me.

Being polite has its place, and it's gotten me far. But sometimes, you've got to show them you're tired of their nonsense and you want help. It's a delicate balance, one I'm still learning to navigate.

As we wait for the nurse to return, I find myself reflecting on the broader implications of this moment. It's not just about getting this procedure done today. It's about the countless other patients who might not have the ability or energy to fight like this. It's about a system that seems designed to wear you down, to make you give up.

But I can't give up. Not when I'm this close. Not when my future - my life - hangs in the balance.

The nurse returns, a cautious smile on her face. "Mr. Pouhé? We've managed to fit you in. It'll be a bit of a wait, but we'll get your procedure done today."

Relief washes over me, so intense it's almost dizzying. "Thank you," I manage to say. "I really appreciate it."

As she leads us back to prepare for the procedure, I make a silent vow. When I'm through this, when I've got my new kidney and my health back, I'm going to find a way to change this system. To make it work better for patients, to make it more humane.

For now, though, I have a heart catheterization to get through. One more hurdle to clear, one step closer to that transplant list. I take a deep breath, squeeze Teri's hand, and follow the nurse down the hall.

The day is just beginning, and I have a feeling it's going to be a long one. But I'm ready. I've been ready for months. And I'm not leaving until I get the answers - and the procedure - I need.

Chapter 17: After the Procedure: A Moment of Relief

The world comes back into focus slowly, like an old television warming up. The stark white ceiling of the recovery room swims above me, and I blink, trying to orient myself. The heart catheterization is over. I made it through.

"Marc? How are you feeling?" Teri's voice comes from somewhere to my left, concern evident in her tone.

I turn my head slightly, careful not to move too much. The doctor's warnings about staying still echo in my mind. "I'm okay," I manage to croak out, my throat dry from the procedure. "What time is it?"

Teri moves into my field of vision, a small smile on her face. "We've been out for about an hour and a half," she says, holding up her phone. "Do you feel up to talking about it? I thought we could record something for your documentary."

I nod slowly, the fog in my mind starting to clear. Teri positions herself off-camera, and I hear the familiar beep of the recording starting.

"Okay, Marc is done," Teri says from behind the camera. "We've been out for about an hour and a half."

I take a deep breath, gathering my thoughts. It's strange, trying to piece together the events of the day. "I don't know if I took my watch off," I begin, realizing how disoriented I still feel. "I don't know what time it is even now."

As I start to recount the procedure, the details come back to me. "The heart cath procedure was one where they were supposed to take a visual look inside my heart," I explain, my voice growing stronger as I speak. "They could have done it either through my neck or they were going to do a groin entry. Neck would have a 45-minute recovery. The groin would have taken 5 to 6 hours to recover."

I can't help but let out a small, wry chuckle. "Just my luck, they chose the groin."

As I speak, I'm struck by the enormity of what's just happened. This procedure, this peek inside my heart, could be the key that unlocks my future. The thought sends a wave of emotion through me, a mix of relief, hope, and lingering anxiety.

"But it all worked out really well in the end," I continue, unable to keep the note of excitement from my voice. "They said I had very clear arteries. I've got to follow up at the end of March and he's going to write a full recommendation that I be placed on the transplant list."

The words hang in the air, their significance almost too much to comprehend. After months of setbacks, delays, and frustrations, this feels like a monumental step forward.

"That hurdle is done," I say, more to myself than to the camera. "I don't want to jinx it, but I think at least by April it should be hopefully approved before the board and on the list. And then we'll go from there and try and get a match or corresponding match with the donor exchange network."

As I continue to talk, recounting the fears and anxieties I felt during the procedure, I'm struck by how vulnerable I feel. It's not just the physical vulnerability of lying here, unable to move much without risking reopening the incision. It's an emotional vulnerability, the realization that I'm one step closer to a transplant, to a new chance at life.

"We're doing the interview this way because I'm not allowed to raise my hand," I explain, trying to inject a bit of humor into the situation. "Apparently if I use my abs, I'm going to open up the incision that's by my groin and possibly bleed out."

Teri lets out a small laugh from behind the camera, and I feel a surge of gratitude for her presence, her unwavering support throughout this ordeal.

"I am doing my best not to make moves," I continue, "even though Teri has made me laugh and jump a couple times. But I'm not blaming Teri, I'm just saying. I'm the one that has a hard time remembering rules."

As I finish speaking, a wave of exhaustion washes over me. The adrenaline of the day is wearing off, leaving behind a bone-deep weariness. But underneath the fatigue, there's a glimmer of something else. Hope. Real, tangible hope.

I turn my head slightly, meeting Teri's eyes behind the camera. "We did it," I say softly, my voice thick with emotion. "We're one step closer."

Teri reaches out, taking my hand in hers. "We are," she agrees, her voice equally emotional. "You did great, Marc."

As we sit there in the recovery room, the beeping of monitors a steady backdrop to our moment of quiet celebration, I find myself reflecting on the journey that's brought me here. The frustrations of the morning seem distant now, overshadowed by the positive outcome of the procedure.

There are still challenges ahead, I know. More tests, more waiting, more hurdles to clear. But for now, in this moment, I allow myself to feel a sense of accomplishment. We've cleared another obstacle. We're moving forward.

And for the first time in a long while, the future doesn't seem quite so daunting. It's out there, waiting for me. A new kidney, a new chance at health, a new chapter of life. And I'm one step closer to reaching it.

As I close my eyes, letting the exhaustion of the day take over, I hold onto that feeling of hope. Tomorrow will bring new challenges, new fights. But today, we've won a significant battle. And that's more than enough for now.

Chapter 18: Wheels of Freedom: Leaving the Hospital

The rhythmic squeak of wheelchair wheels echoes through the hospital corridors as an orderly guides me towards the exit. After hours of lying motionless on my back, this simple movement feels like a luxury. The fluorescent lights overhead create a strobe effect as we pass beneath them, each flash a reminder that I'm one step closer to home.

"Alright, thank you," I say to the orderly, gratitude welling up inside me. It's not just for the ride to the exit, but for everything - the care, the successful procedure, the chance to move forward.

The orderly's voice is warm, genuinely pleased. "Glad you're going home."

"Me too, man," I respond, unable to keep a note of wry humor from my voice. "Six hours on my back was a unique experience. Not as unique as using the bedpan twice for the first time in my life."

As soon as the words leave my mouth, I feel a twinge of embarrassment. But the orderly doesn't miss a beat.

"All normal," he assures me, his tone matter-of-fact and free of judgment.

His simple acceptance eases my discomfort, reminding me that in a hospital, these things are indeed just part of the routine. "It's completely normal as long as you're-" I begin, but he cuts me off gently.

"You're good. You're going home."

Those words - "You're going home" - hit me with unexpected force. I'm going home. Away from the constant beeping of monitors, the smell of disinfectant, the perpetual state of vulnerability that comes with being a patient. I'm going back to my own space, my own bed, a semblance of normalcy.

"I tell you," I continue, feeling a need to process this experience out loud, "the second time was a lot more normal than the first time."

The orderly's response is a mixture of professionalism and human understanding. "Yes, hey we're all used to it. We're in it."

His words strike me as profound in their simplicity. They're in it - day in, day out, dealing with the messy, uncomfortable realities of human bodies and human vulnerability. I feel a surge of appreciation for this often-overlooked aspect of healthcare.

"That's good. You guys are trained professionals, man. I appreciate that," I tell him, trying to convey the depth of my gratitude in these simple words.

"Of course. We try to be," he responds humbly. Then, with a philosophical tone that catches me off guard, he adds, "It could always be worse, oh but it's such a blessing."

As we approach the hospital exit, his words echo in my mind. It could always be worse, but it's such a blessing. Isn't that the essence of my entire journey? The constant balance between acknowledging the difficulties and being grateful for the progress, the care, the chance at a better future?

The automatic doors slide open, and a gust of fresh air hits me. It's invigorating after hours in the climate-controlled hospital environment. Teri is there, pulling up in our car, a smile of relief on her face.

As the orderly helps me into the passenger seat, I'm overwhelmed by a mix of emotions. Relief at leaving the hospital, gratitude for the care I've received, anxiety about the road ahead, hope for what this successful procedure might mean for my transplant prospects.

"Thank you," I say again to the orderly as he closes the car door. "For everything."

He gives me a nod and a smile. "Take care of yourself."

As Teri pulls away from the curb, I watch the hospital recede in the side mirror. This building, with its maze of corridors and rooms, has been the site of so many pivotal moments in my journey. Fear, pain, frustration, but also hope, progress, and now, potentially, a major step towards my ultimate goal.

"How are you feeling?" Teri asks, reaching over to squeeze my hand.

I take a moment to really consider her question. How am I feeling? Tired, certainly. Sore from lying in one position for so long. A bit apprehensive about the incision site and the need to be careful in the coming days.

But underneath all that, there's something else. A quiet sense of accomplishment, of forward momentum.

"I'm feeling... hopeful," I finally respond. "We did it, Teri. We got through this. And now..."

"And now we wait for the results and the recommendation," she finishes for me.

I nod, letting out a long breath. "Yeah. More waiting. But this time, it feels different. Like we're waiting for good news, you know?"

As we drive home through the familiar streets of our town, I find myself reflecting on the orderly's words again. It could always be worse, but it's such a blessing. Yes, there's more waiting ahead. Yes, there are still hurdles to overcome. But today, we cleared a major one. Today, we moved one step closer to the transplant list, to a new kidney, to a new lease on life.

I lean my head back against the headrest, allowing myself to really feel the weight of today's accomplishment. The fear I felt this morning, the frustration with the scheduling issues, the discomfort of the procedure itself - it all seems worth it now.

As our house comes into view, I feel a sense of peace settle over me. We're home. We made it through. And tomorrow, we'll face whatever comes next.

For now, though, I'm content to bask in this moment of quiet triumph. One more hurdle cleared. One step closer to a new beginning.

Chapter 19: Bridging Distances: A Father-Daughter Moment

The familiar chime of an incoming Zoom call breaks the quiet of my Sunday morning. I settle into my chair, adjusting the laptop screen as Angelina's face comes into focus. At 17, she's a young woman now, her features a perfect blend of her mother and me. The sight of her sends a pang through my heart - a mixture of pride, love, and a touch of regret for the time and distance that separates us.

"Hey, Dad," she says, her smile brightening the screen. "How are you feeling?"

The genuine concern in her voice touches me deeply. I've tried to shield my children from the worst of my health struggles, but they're old enough now to understand the gravity of the situation. "I'm doing okay, sweetheart," I respond, mustering a smile of my own. "Better every day."

We chat for a while about her school, her friends, her plans for the future. With each passing minute, I'm struck by how articulate and thoughtful she's become. It seems like just yesterday she was a little girl, and now here she is, on the cusp of adulthood, with opinions and dreams all her own.

"You know," I say, a note of wistfulness creeping into my voice, "you outsmarted me maybe five or six years ago. You're 17 now and I'm just proud of everything you do and I look forward to your future."

Angelina laughs, a sound that warms me from the inside out. "Dad, stop," she says, but I can see the pleased flush in her cheeks.

I glance at the time, aware that I still need to take my morning medicine. "Anything else you want to talk about before we get off?" I ask, not wanting to cut our time short but mindful of my health routine.

Angelina's eyes light up, and I can almost see the gears turning in her mind. "Well," she begins, "one thing I did want to talk about is when you think about the electoral college system, when you think about the foundations of the country..."

What follows is a detailed, passionate explanation of her views on democracy, representation, and the need for systemic change. I listen, captivated not just by her words, but by the fire behind them. This is my daughter, I think with a surge of pride. This brilliant, engaged, compassionate young woman.

As she speaks, I'm struck by the contrast between her world and mine. Here I am, my days revolving around dialysis schedules and doctor's appointments, while she's out there, her mind grappling with big ideas, her heart set on changing the world. There's a bittersweetness to it - a reminder of the life I've stepped back from, but also a profound gratitude that she's able to pursue her passions so vigorously.

When she finally pauses for breath, I nod, a smile playing at the corners of my mouth. "I agree," I say. "I definitely agree."

For a moment, we just look at each other, and I'm acutely aware of how precious these moments are. How easily they could have been lost if things had gone differently with my health.

"Well, it's been a real pleasure talking with you today," I say, trying to keep my voice steady despite the emotion welling up inside me. "I hope you have a good rest of your Sunday and enjoy your spring break. I love you."

"Love you too, Dad," Angelina replies. "Bye."

As the call ends and her face disappears from my screen, I sit back in my chair, letting out a long breath. These conversations with my children are always a mix of joy and melancholy. Joy at seeing them grow, develop their own thoughts and personalities. Melancholy at the physical distance between us, at the time lost to my illness.

I think about the journey I'm on - the dialysis, the constant medical appointments, the recent heart catheterization. It's all aimed at one goal: to be there for moments like these. To watch my children grow, to be part of their lives, to see the amazing adults they're becoming.

As I reach for my morning medications, I'm filled with a renewed sense of purpose. Every pill swallowed, every procedure endured, every hurdle overcome - it's all for this. For the chance to be a father to Angelina and her siblings, to be present in their lives, to see where their bright minds and big hearts will take them.

The road ahead is still long and uncertain. The transplant list, the wait for a donor, the surgery itself - there are still many challenges to face. But conversations like this one with Angelina remind me why it's all worth it. They give me strength to face whatever comes next.

I swallow my pills, my mind still full of Angelina's words about democracy and change. My daughter, the future activist, the thinker, the doer. Whatever happens with my health, I realize, a part of me will live on through her and her siblings - through their ideas, their passions, their determination to make the world a better place.

With that thought warming me, I stand up, ready to face the rest of my day. There's dialysis to prepare for, doctor's instructions to follow, a delicate balance of rest and activity to maintain. But now, more than ever, I'm reminded of why I'm fighting so hard. For moments like these. For the future. For family.

Chapter 20: The Verdict: A Step Closer to New Life

The familiar scent of disinfectant greets me as I step into the cardiologist's office. It's a smell I've become intimately acquainted with over the past months, but today it carries a different weight. Today, I'm here for more than just another check-up. Today could be the day that changes everything.

As I settle into the waiting room chair, I can feel my heart racing, a rapid staccato that seems to echo in my ears. The irony isn't lost on me - here I am, in a cardiologist's office, my heart working overtime due to nerves rather than medical issues.

"Mr. Pouhé?" A nurse calls my name, and I stand, following her down the corridor to the examination room. Each step feels monumental, as if I'm walking towards a future that's still undefined, still hanging in the balance.

The Physician's Assistant enters, a warm smile on her face. "Hey, how are you doing?" she asks, her tone friendly and familiar.

"I'm fantastic," I respond, surprising myself with the enthusiasm in my voice. Despite the nerves, there's an undercurrent of hope that I can't suppress.

She glances down at my chart, her eyebrows rising slightly. "It looks like you've got clean coronaries," she begins, and I feel my breath catch in my throat. "And interestingly, did the doctor talk to you after the heart cath? Did he tell you that we didn't see any evidence of a stent?"

"How strange," I manage to say, my mind whirling. No stent? But I was so sure... The memory of that long-ago hospital visit in 2009 flashes through my mind, the fear and pain of that time suddenly vivid again.

The PA continues her examination, asking about my symptoms, my dialysis schedule. I answer automatically, my thoughts still caught on the revelation about the missing stent. It's as if a piece of my medical history, a part of my identity as a patient, has suddenly been called into question.

As we talk, I find myself marveling at how far I've come. From that scared man in 2009, facing a health crisis he barely understood, to now - on the cusp of a potential transplant, navigating the complex world of specialized medical care with a knowledge born of hard experience.

The door opens again, and Dr. Heustlein enters. His presence fills the small room, and I feel a mix of respect and apprehension. This man holds my future in his hands.

"Hey, how are you doing?" he asks, his voice carrying the confident authority of someone used to delivering life-changing news, both good and bad.

"I'm good, how are you?" I respond, trying to keep my voice steady.

Dr. Heustlein doesn't waste time on small talk. "Alright. I don't even know. Oh, I guess we had to do this. We could officially put it in writing. You are crystal clear for transplant."

The words hit me like a physical force. Crystal clear for transplant. I've been hoping for this, working towards this, but to hear it stated so plainly... It's overwhelming.

"You had beautiful arteries," Dr. Heustlein continues, his voice taking on an almost admiring tone. "I don't know. I guess there was somebody that said they put a stent in you or something at some point. I thought I was going to find a stent."

As he speaks, explaining about bioresorbable stents and the pristine condition of my arteries, I find myself transported back in time. To sleepless nights worrying about my heart health, to the fear that my cardiac issues might disqualify me from transplant. And now, to hear that not only am I cleared, but that my arteries are "beautiful"... It's almost too much to process.

"Now, there might have been one that was there," Dr. Heustlein is saying. "They have these things now they're called bioresorbable. I don't know if they had them in 2009, they don't leave any visible markers but if they put one in, they did a beautiful job and your arteries are pristine."

I nod, trying to take it all in. The mystery of the missing stent, the unexpected good news about my cardiac health - it's a lot to process. But underneath it all is a growing sense of elation. I'm cleared. I'm one giant step closer to transplant.

As Dr. Heustlein continues to explain the results, I find my thoughts racing ahead. What does this mean for my place on the transplant list? How soon could it happen? The possibilities seem to stretch out before me, a future that suddenly feels more tangible than it has in years.

"Well, best of luck to you," Dr. Heustlein says, wrapping up the appointment. "Enjoy the new kidney."

The casual way he says it - "enjoy the new kidney" - as if it's a foregone conclusion, hits me hard. For so long, the transplant has been a distant hope, a maybe. But now, in Dr. Heustlein's matter-of-fact tone, it feels real. Possible. Imminent, even.

"Alright, thanks a lot, sir," I manage to say, my voice thick with emotion.

"Makes life better," he adds as he heads for the door.

"Have a great day," I call after him.

"You too," he responds. "And you don't need to check out, do a follow-up, do anything, you're good to go."

As the door closes behind him, I sit for a moment, letting it all sink in. Good to go. Cleared for transplant. Beautiful arteries. The words swirl in my mind, each one a stepping stone towards a future I've been fighting so hard to reach.

I stand slowly, gathering my things. As I step out of the examination room, the world seems different somehow. Brighter. Full of possibility. The other patients in the waiting room, the nurses at their stations - they have no idea that my life has just changed dramatically. That I've just received the news I've been hoping for, praying for, for so long.

As I walk out of the office and into the sunlight, I take a deep breath. The air seems fresher somehow, the colors more vibrant. I'm cleared for transplant. I'm one step closer to a new kidney, to a new life.

There's still a long road ahead, I know. Waiting lists, more tests, the surgery itself, recovery. But for now, in this moment, I allow myself to feel the full weight of this victory. To savor it. To let hope, real and tangible, fill me up.

I pull out my phone, eager to share the news with Teri, with my kids, with everyone who's been on this journey with me. But for a moment, I just stand there, letting the sun warm my face, letting the reality of it all wash over me.

I'm cleared for transplant. I'm moving forward. And for the first time in a long time, the future looks bright indeed.

Chapter 21: Listening to the Body

The sterile smell of the examination room fills my nostrils as I sit across from Dr. Gentry, my new nephrologist. It's become a familiar scent, one that no longer triggers the anxiety it once did. Instead, it's almost comforting in its familiarity, a reminder of the journey I'm on.

"So, Marc," Dr. Gentry begins, her voice warm but professional, "how have you been feeling since our last appointment?"

I take a deep breath, mentally cataloging the various aches, pains, and changes I've noticed over the past weeks. It's become second nature now, this hyper-awareness of my body's every twinge and shift.

"Well," I start, "I've been having some issues with urination lately." The words come out matter-of-factly, a stark contrast to how I might have approached such a topic in the past.

As I describe my symptoms, I can't help but marvel at how different this experience is from my younger days. There was a time when I barely paid attention to my body's signals, when I pushed through discomfort and ignored warning signs. Now, every change is noted, analyzed, reported.

Dr. Gentry listens intently, her brow furrowing slightly as I speak. When I finish, she nods thoughtfully. "I think we should have you see a urologist," she says. "These symptoms warrant further investigation."

As she writes out the referral, my mind drifts back to 2011, to a memory that still fills me with a mix of shock and shame. I had been in the hospital, feeling generally unwell but unable to pinpoint exactly why. A nurse had approached me, asking for a urine sample.

It was in that moment, faced with such a simple request, that the horrifying realization hit me: I couldn't provide a sample. I hadn't urinated in... how long? Days? Weeks? The fact that I couldn't even remember when I had last urinated was a stark testament to how disconnected I had been from my own body.

The memory of that younger, sicker version of myself stands in sharp contrast to who I am now. That man had been so consumed by his illness, so overwhelmed by the daily struggle of survival, that he had failed to notice when his kidneys completely shut down. Now, years later, I find myself hyper-aware of every bodily function, every small change a potential harbinger of new challenges.

"Marc?" Dr. Gentry's voice pulls me back to the present. "Are you alright?"

I nod, blinking away the remnants of the memory. "Yes, sorry. Just... remembering something."

She gives me a sympathetic smile. "This journey isn't just physical, is it? There's a lot of emotional territory to navigate as well."

Her words hit home, and I feel a sudden wave of gratitude for her understanding. "You're right," I admit. "Sometimes it feels like I'm constantly reliving parts of my medical history, comparing then and now."

"That's completely normal," she assures me. "You've been through a lot, and you're still going through a lot. It's natural to reflect on how far you've come."

As I leave her office, referral in hand, I'm struck by the dual nature of my current situation. On one hand, I'm dealing with a new health concern, another potential obstacle on my path to transplant. On the other hand, the very fact that I noticed these symptoms, that I'm actively seeking answers, is a testament to how far I've come.

The urologist, Dr. Patel, turns out to be a stark contrast to my experiences with other specialists. Where getting an appointment with the cardiologist had been an exercise in patience and persistence, Dr. Patel's office seems eager to see me. Appointments are scheduled, then moved up. It's almost disconcerting how quickly things are moving.

Over the course of several weeks, Dr. Patel puts me through a battery of tests. Each one is explained in detail, my questions answered with patience and clarity. It's a refreshing change from the often opaque world of medical procedures I've become accustomed to.

Finally, Dr. Patel calls me in to discuss the results. As I sit in his office, I can feel my heart racing, a familiar anxiety bubbling up despite my best efforts to remain calm.

"Well, Mr. Pouhé," he begins, his tone serious but not alarming, "we've identified the issue. You're experiencing prostate enlargement, likely age-related."

The diagnosis hits me with a mix of relief and concern. Relief that we've identified the problem, concern about what it might mean for my overall health and my chances for transplant.

"The good news," Dr. Patel continues, "is that we can treat this. I recommend a HoLEP surgery - that's a laser procedure that should provide a permanent solution."

As he explains the details of the surgery, I find myself marveling at how far medical technology has come. A laser to treat prostate enlargement? It sounds like science fiction. Yet here I am, discussing it as casually as if we were talking about a routine check-up.

The surgery itself goes smoothly, and for a while, it seems like the issue has been resolved. But about two months later, the difficulty urinating returns. The speed with which Dr. Patel diagnoses the issue this time is almost dizzying.

"It appears you've developed some internal scarring," he explains during our follow-up. "It's not common, but it can happen. We'll need to do the procedure again, but this time, we'll inject steroids to prevent further scarring."

The prospect of another surgery is daunting, but I appreciate Dr. Patel's proactive approach. This time, the recovery includes a week with a Foley catheter - an experience that's uncomfortable but manageable, especially compared to some of the other medical challenges I've faced.

As I recover from the second surgery, I find myself reflecting on the complex journey my body has taken me on. From the young man so disconnected from his physical self that he didn't notice when his kidneys failed, to the hyper-vigilant patient I've become, analyzing every symptom, every change.

The steroids do their job, unlike my experience with prednisone back in 2009 - a chapter of my medical history I'm not quite ready to revisit. This time, the treatment works as intended, resolving the urinary issues without the devastating side effects I had experienced in the past.

As I share the outcome of the surgeries with Dr. Gentry during our next appointment, I can't help but feel a sense of accomplishment. It's not just that we've successfully addressed the prostate issue. It's the realization of how far I've come in advocating for my own health, in being an active participant in my medical care rather than a passive recipient.

"You've handled this remarkably well," Dr. Gentry comments, a note of approval in her voice. "It's not easy dealing with additional health issues while waiting for a transplant."

I nod, feeling a mix of pride and weariness. "It's been a journey," I admit. "Sometimes it feels like my body is a puzzle, and we're constantly discovering new pieces."

Dr. Gentry smiles sympathetically. "That's not a bad way to look at it. The important thing is that you're paying attention, you're advocating for yourself. That's crucial, especially as we continue to work towards transplant."

As I leave her office that day, I feel a renewed sense of determination. Yes, my body continues to present new challenges. Yes, the road to transplant is long and uncertain. But I'm no longer that disconnected young man, oblivious to the signals my body was sending. I've become an active participant in my own health journey, a collaborator with my medical team rather than just a patient.

The urological issues have been a detour on my path to transplant, but they've also been a reminder of my resilience, of my capacity to face new challenges head-on. As I prepare for my nightly dialysis, I find myself looking forward to the future with cautious optimism.

I settle into my dialysis chair, the familiar hum of the machine a backdrop to my thoughts. As I watch my blood flow through the tubes, cleansing and returning, I'm struck by a profound realization. This body of mine, with all its complexities and challenges, is not my enemy. It's my partner in this journey, constantly communicating, constantly adapting.

Whatever new puzzles my body might present, I'm ready to face them, one piece at a time. Because each challenge overcome, each hurdle cleared, brings me one step closer to that ultimate goal: a new kidney, a new chance at health, a new chapter in this ongoing story of survival and hope.

Chapter 22: The Waiting Game

The soft glow of my phone screen illuminates the pre-dawn darkness of my bedroom. It's become a ritual, this early morning check – Is it charged? Is the volume on? Have I missed any calls? My heart races a little, as it does every morning, at the possibility that today could be the day. The day that changes everything.

As I carefully unplug my phone and set it on the nightstand, I'm acutely aware of the dichotomy of my existence. On one hand, my life has settled into a routine defined by dialysis schedules and medication regimens. On the other, I live in a constant state of anticipation, knowing that at any moment, day or night, I could receive the call that would catapult me into a new chapter of my life.

I ease myself out of bed, mindful of the catheter site as I stand. The house is quiet, Teri still asleep. In these early morning hours, the weight of waiting feels particularly heavy. I make my way to the kitchen, the familiar path now easily navigated even in the dim light.

As I wait for the coffee to brew, I find myself rehearsing the conversation I've had countless times in my head. "Hello, this is the transplant center. We have a kidney for you." How would I react? Would I be calm and collected, or would the emotion of the moment overwhelm me?

The coffee maker gurgles its last, pulling me from my reverie. As I pour my first cup, careful to stay within my strict fluid restrictions, I glance at the calendar on the fridge. Another day to cross off. Another day of waiting.

Later that morning, as I settle in for my regular check-in call with the transplant center, I feel the familiar mix of hope and anxiety bubbling up.

"Any updates on my status?" I ask, trying to keep my voice casual. "Or... on the potential living donor?"

The coordinator's voice is gentle but neutral, a tone I've become all too familiar with. "Your status remains active on the deceased donor list. As for the living donor, they're progressing through their evaluation process. These things take time, Marc. It's thorough for a reason."

I nod, forgetting for a moment that she can't see me. "I understand," I say, hoping my disappointment isn't too evident in my voice. "Thank you for the update."

As I hang up, I'm struck by the strange limbo I find myself in. The thoroughness of the process is something I understand all too well. Every test, every evaluation, is a safeguard – not just for me, but for the potential donor as well. Yet the waiting, the not knowing, sometimes feels like a form of torture.

My phone pings with a notification. It's a message from the potential donor, their updates a mix of medical details and personal reflections that have become a bright spot in this often-grueling waiting game.

"Another round of tests today. The nurses were so kind. Feeling good about this!"

Their enthusiasm is infectious, a reminder of the incredible generosity that underlies their actions. Yet, as I read their message, I feel the familiar twinge of guilt. How much should I share of my own journey? The recent urological issues, the constant balancing act of managing my health – it all feels like too much to burden them with.

That evening, as I prepare for dialysis, I find myself composing a message to them:

"Your updates mean more to me than I can express. I'm in awe of your kindness and determination. My own journey has had some unexpected turns lately, but knowing you're out there, going through this process for me, gives me strength. Thank you doesn't seem enough, but thank you."

My finger hovers over the send button for a long moment before I finally press it. It feels like a small step, an acknowledgment of their importance in my life, a tiny window into my experience without overwhelming them with the full weight of my struggles.

Their response comes quickly: "I'm here for you, whatever turns your journey takes. We're in this together, even if our paths look different."

Their words bring a lump to my throat. In this moment, the waiting feels a little less lonely, the future a little brighter.

As the weeks turn into months, I find the transplant process beginning to feel less like a sprint and more like a marathon. The initial adrenaline of being listed has given way to a steadier, more measured approach to waiting. It's during one of my regular check-ups with Dr. Gentry that I realize just how much this waiting period has affected me.

"How are you holding up, Marc?" she asks, her eyes searching my face with the keen insight I've come to appreciate.

I sigh, running a hand over my head. "It's... challenging," I admit, the words feeling inadequate to express the complexity of emotions I'm grappling with. "Some days, the wait feels endless. Other days, I'm terrified I'm not ready."

She nods, understanding evident in her expression. "That's normal. This waiting period isn't just about physical preparation. It's mental and emotional preparation too."

Her words strike a chord, resonating deeply. I realize that each health challenge I've faced – from the billing disputes to the urological issues – has been preparing me in its own way.

Each obstacle overcome is another step towards being ready for the transplant, whenever it might come.

As summer turns to fall, I receive news that sends a jolt through my carefully cultivated equilibrium. The transplant coordinator calls, her voice tinged with an excitement I've never heard before.

"Marc, I have an update for you. Your potential living donor has completed their initial evaluation process successfully. We're moving forward to the next phase."

The news hits me like a wave, a mixture of hope and anxiety washing over me. This is progress, tangible progress towards a possible transplant. Yet it also brings the reality of what lies ahead into sharp focus.

In the days that follow, I find myself reflecting on the journey that has brought me to this point. The years of declining health, the nightly dialysis, the constant battle with insurance and medical bills – it all seems to culminate in this moment of possibility.

I think about the person who has volunteered to be my donor, someone willing to undergo major surgery to give me a chance at a better life. Their generosity is a constant reminder of the good in the world, a counterbalance to the often frustrating and dehumanizing aspects of the healthcare system I've been battling.

Yet, as the possibility of transplant becomes more real, so do the fears. What if something goes wrong? What if my body rejects the kidney? What if, after all this, I can't live up to the gift I'm being given?

During my next dialysis session, I share these fears with Teri. Her hand finds mine, a gesture of comfort we've perfected over countless nights like this.

"It's okay to be scared," she says softly, her voice barely audible over the hum of the dialysis machine. "But remember how far you've come. You've faced every challenge head-on. This is just the next step."

Her words, as always, are a balm to my anxious mind. I realize that the waiting, as difficult as it has been, has also been a gift in its own way. It has given me time to grow stronger, both physically and mentally. It has allowed me to face and overcome other health challenges, making me more resilient for what lies ahead.

As the dialysis machine hums its familiar tune, I find myself feeling a cautious optimism. The road ahead is still uncertain, filled with potential challenges and unknowns. But for the first time in a long while, it also feels filled with real possibility.

The waiting game isn't over. In many ways, it's entering a new, more intense phase. But as I sit here, connected to the machine that has become such a huge part of my life, I feel ready. Ready to face whatever comes next, be it more waiting, more challenges, or finally, the transplant itself.

The journey has changed me, shaped me in ways I'm only beginning to understand. And whatever the future holds, I know I will face it with the strength and resilience I have found along the way. The wait continues, but now it's tinged with hope – hope for a new kidney, yes, but also hope for a future where I can live fully, free from the constraints of dialysis and chronic illness.

As the session ends and I disconnect from the machine, I feel a sense of determination settle over me. Tomorrow is another day of waiting, but it's also another day closer to the possibility of a new life. And for now, that possibility is enough to keep me going, one day at a time.

I reach for my phone, opening the camera app that has become my constant companion on this journey. "Another day down," I say to the lens, my voice low but steady. "Another day closer to whatever comes next. I don't know what tomorrow will bring, but I know I'm ready for it. This waiting game... it's tough. But it's also teaching me patience, resilience, and gratitude in ways I never expected."

I pause, considering my next words carefully. "To anyone out there waiting – for a transplant, for healing, for any kind of life-changing moment – I see you. I feel your struggle.

And I hope you can find strength in the waiting, just as I'm trying to do. We're all in this together, even when it feels most isolating."

As I end the recording, I feel a sense of connection to the broader community of patients and caregivers who are on similar journeys. The waiting game is universal, I realize. And in sharing my story, in documenting this journey, I'm not just processing my own experiences – I'm potentially providing a lifeline to others who might be feeling just as lost, just as scared, just as hopeful as I am.

With that thought, I turn off the light and head to bed. Tomorrow is another day of waiting, yes. But it's also another day of living, of growing, of moving forward – one small step at a time.

Chapter 23: The Gift and The Wait

The vibration of my phone against the kitchen counter sends a jolt through my body. It's a Tuesday afternoon, and I'm in the middle of preparing my afternoon medications when the transplant coordinator's number flashes on the screen. My heart leaps into my throat as I reach for the device, my hand trembling slightly. Is this the call? The one we've been waiting for?

"Hello?" My voice comes out as a croak, and I clear my throat, trying to sound more composed than I feel.

"Marc," the coordinator's voice is warm, excited even. "I have some significant updates for you. Your living donor has completed the entire evaluation process successfully."

A tidal wave of emotion crashes over me – gratitude, hope, excitement. The room seems to spin for a moment, and I grip the counter for support. But before I can fully process these feelings, the coordinator continues, her tone shifting slightly.

"However, I need to explain something important. You and your donor aren't a perfect match."

My heart plummets, the brief moment of elation giving way to a familiar disappointment. But she quickly adds, "But this isn't bad news. Far from it. Your donor's willingness to donate on your behalf significantly improves your position on both the living and deceased donor lists."

As she launches into an explanation of the modern kidney exchange program, I find myself sinking into a kitchen chair, my legs suddenly weak. My mind races back to 2012, to my brother's donation. I remember the agonizing wait as we tried to align six people – three donors, three recipients – like some bizarre medical jigsaw puzzle.

"The current system prioritizes donors," the coordinator explains, her voice pulling me back to the present. "It gives them more flexibility in scheduling their surgeries. This is great for donor retention and can speed up the process overall."

I nod, even though she can't see me. It makes sense – anything that makes the process easier for donors can only be a good thing. These are people volunteering to undergo major surgery to help others, after all. The magnitude of their generosity never ceases to amaze me.

"So what does this mean for me?" I ask, unable to keep a tremor of anxiety from my voice. Hope and fear wage a silent war in my chest as I wait for her response.

"It means you're in a much better position now," she replies, her tone reassuring. "But – and I need you to understand this – you still need to wait for your perfect match. Your donor may be able to donate to someone else before you receive your kidney."

The implications of this hit me like a physical blow. The person who had so generously stepped forward to help me might end up helping someone else instead. It's a beautiful thing, really – a chain of kindness extending beyond just me. But it also means more waiting, more uncertainty. The familiar weight of anticipation settles back onto my shoulders, heavier than before.

As the days pass, I find myself grappling with a complex mix of emotions. Overwhelming gratitude for my donor's selflessness. Hope that my perfect match will come soon. And, if I'm being honest, a gnawing frustration that I can't seem to shake. When will it be my turn?

During one of my dialysis sessions, I share these feelings with Teri. The steady hum of the machine provides a backdrop to our conversation, a constant reminder of why this matters so much.

"I feel guilty even thinking it," I admit, my voice barely above a whisper. "Someone is giving a huge gift, and here I am, feeling impatient."

Teri squeezes my hand, her touch warm and comforting against my skin. "It's okay to feel that way," she says softly, her eyes meeting mine with understanding. "This isn't an easy journey. Your feelings are valid."

Her understanding helps, but the internal struggle continues. I'm deeply grateful for my donor's gift, even if it might not directly benefit me. Their willingness to donate has significantly improved my chances. But the waiting, the constant state of limbo, is wearing on me in ways I hadn't anticipated.

One evening, as I'm preparing for dialysis, meticulously laying out my supplies with the precision born of long practice, my phone chimes. It's a message from my donor. My heart races as I open it, wondering what news it might bring.

"Just got word – I'm scheduled for surgery next month! So excited to be able to help someone."

Their enthusiasm is palpable, their kindness overwhelming. I feel a swell of emotions – joy for them, gratitude for their generosity, and yes, a twinge of envy that I immediately feel ashamed of. They're moving forward, while I remain in waiting.

I stare at my phone for a long moment, carefully crafting my response. The words need to be perfect, need to convey the depth of my gratitude while hiding the complex swirl of emotions their news has stirred up.

"That's wonderful news!" I type, pausing between each word. "I'm so happy for you, and for the person who will receive your incredible gift. Your kindness has already made a huge difference in my life, improving my chances for a match. Thank you doesn't seem enough, but thank you, from the bottom of my heart."

As I hit send, I feel a mix of genuine happiness for them and a renewed determination to stay positive in my own journey. Their gift, even if not directly to me, is part of a larger network of kindness and hope. It's making a difference, setting off a chain reaction that will help not just one person, but potentially many.

The days continue to pass, each one a mix of hope and resignation. I remain active on both the living and deceased donor lists, my position improved thanks to my donor's generosity. But still, the perfect match remains elusive. Each day begins with a moment of anticipation as I check my phone, and ends with a small sigh of disappointment when no news comes.

During a check-up with Dr. Gentry, she notices my subdued mood. Her eyes, kind but scrutinizing, search my face as she asks, "How are you holding up, Marc?"

I sigh, running a hand over my face, feeling the fatigue etched into every line. "I'm grateful, I really am," I begin, struggling to find the right words. "But... I can't help wondering, when will it be my turn? Am I wrong to feel this way?"

Dr. Gentry's eyes are kind as she replies, her voice carrying the weight of years of experience with patients in similar situations. "It's not wrong at all. This process is challenging, emotionally as well as physically. It's okay to acknowledge that."

Her validation helps, reminding me that it's okay to have complex, even contradictory feelings about this journey. Gratitude and frustration can coexist. Hope and impatience are not mutually exclusive.

As the date of my donor's surgery approaches, I find myself reflecting on the journey that has brought me to this point. The years of declining health, the nightly dialysis, the constant battle with the healthcare system – it has all led to this moment of continued waiting, but with a new perspective.

I think about the person who volunteered to be my donor, someone willing to undergo major surgery to give a stranger a chance at a better life. Their generosity is a constant reminder of the good in the world, a counterbalance to the often frustrating and dehumanizing aspects of the healthcare system I have been battling.

The day of their surgery, I send them a message of support and gratitude. As I hit send, I realize that this journey has taught me something profound about the nature of giving and receiving. Sometimes, the greatest gifts we receive aren't the ones given directly to us, but the ones that inspire hope, kindness, and a sense of connection to a larger community of caring individuals.

As I settle in for another night of dialysis, the familiar hum of the machine a soundtrack to my thoughts, I find myself feeling a complex mix of emotions. Gratitude for my donor's selflessness. Hope for the future, knowing that my chances for a match have improved. Frustration at the continued wait. And underneath it all, a steely determination to keep going, to stay strong for whatever lies ahead.

I reach for my phone, opening the camera app that has become my confidant throughout this journey. The lens captures my face, the lines of fatigue etched around my eyes, but also the glimmer of hope that I can feel burning within me.

"Another day," I say to the camera, my voice low but steady. "Another day of waiting, but also another day of living. This gift, even if it's not directly to me, has changed everything. It's a reminder of the goodness in the world, of the power of human kindness."

I pause, gathering my thoughts. "The wait continues, but so does hope. And that's something worth holding onto."

As I end the recording, I realize that this chapter of my story – our story – doesn't have an immediate happy ending. I'm still waiting for my perfect kidney, still navigating the challenges of life on dialysis. But it's a story of resilience, of the power of human kindness, and of the complex journey of learning to receive as well as to give.

The dialysis machine continues its work, the steady rhythm a reminder of both my current reality and the hope for a different future. I close my eyes and allow myself to imagine a world beyond this waiting. A future made possible by the kindness of strangers, the advances of medical science, and my own determination to keep fighting, keep hoping, keep living.

The wait continues, but so does my story. And for now, that is enough. One day at a time, one step at a time, I will keep moving forward, carrying with me the strength I have found in this journey and the incredible gift of human kindness that has already changed my life in ways I am only beginning to understand.

As I drift off to sleep, the dialysis machine humming softly in the background, I hold onto that spark of hope. Tomorrow is another day of waiting, yes. But it's also another day closer to the possibility of a new life. And that possibility, that hope, is what keeps me going, one day at a time.

Chapter 24: The Call and The Promise: A New Chapter Begins

The soft chime of my phone cuts through the quiet of my home office. I glance at the screen, my heart skipping a beat as I read the caller ID: Abdominal Transplant. My hand trembles slightly as I reach for the device, a mixture of hope and anxiety coursing through me.

"Hello?" I answer, trying to keep my voice steady.

"Hi, is this Marc?" A friendly female voice comes through the speaker.

"This is Marc," I confirm, my free hand gripping the edge of my desk.

"Hey Marc. It's Katie, I'm returning your phone call."

I let out a small chuckle, some of the tension easing from my shoulders. "Hey Katie. Playing phone tag."

"Oh no, it's-" she starts, then seems to change course. "Hey, I just want to let you know your donor has been made active in the National Kidney Registry system."

The words hit me like a physical force. Active in the system. It's really happening. I lean back in my chair, closing my eyes for a moment as I try to process this information.

Katie continues, her voice excited but professional. "Hopefully we'll get a date when she can donate. The next steps for you, once she donates, I can make you active in the system as long as we have everything we need, and the only thing we're missing is a cheek swab that needs to be done."

As she explains the process and next steps, I find myself only half-listening, my mind racing ahead. This is it. The moment we've been waiting for, hoping for, praying for. It's finally within reach.

"Well, thank you, I appreciate it," I manage to say when she finishes, my voice thick with emotion.

"You're welcome, Marc. Take care and hopefully we'll talk soon."

We exchange goodbyes, and as I hang up the phone, I'm overwhelmed by a wave of emotions. Joy, gratitude, anxiety, hope - they all swirl together, leaving me breathless.

I stand up, needing to move, to do something with this excess energy suddenly coursing through me. I pace the length of my office, my mind whirling with the implications of this call.

"Things are moving quickly," I say aloud, the sound of my own voice grounding me in the moment. "I have a donor who is already set up to donate."

I pause, running a hand through my hair as I try to organize my thoughts. The system, the process - it's all so complex, so intricate. "But the way the system works," I continue, speaking to the empty room as if trying to make sense of it all, "is my donor can donate at a time that's convenient for them."

This thought brings a fresh wave of emotions. The generosity of my donor, their willingness to go through major surgery for me - it's almost too much to comprehend. And yet, there's also a twinge of anxiety. What if their convenient time is weeks or months from now? How much longer will I have to wait?

I shake my head, pushing away these thoughts. No, I remind myself. This is a moment for gratitude, for hope. Whatever happens next, this is a huge step forward.

I sink back into my chair, suddenly exhausted. The weight of this moment, the potential it holds for my future, settles over me like a heavy blanket. I reach for my phone again, this time opening the camera app.

"Just got off the phone with the transplant center," I say to the lens, my voice steadier now. "Things are moving forward. My donor is active in the system. It's... it's really happening."

I pause, swallowing hard against the lump in my throat. "I don't know what comes next, or how long it will take. But this... this is the closest we've been. It's real now."

As I end the recording, I'm struck by how much has changed in the past few months. From the depths of illness to this moment of hope - it's been a journey I never could have imagined.

I close my eyes, allowing myself a moment to simply breathe, to exist in this space of possibility. Tomorrow will bring new challenges, new worries. But for now, in this moment, I let myself feel the full weight of this gift I've been given. The gift of hope, of a future that suddenly seems so much brighter.

Whatever comes next, I know I'm ready. Ready to face the challenges, ready to embrace the possibilities. Ready to take this next step on the long road to healing.

As the afternoon sun streams through my office window, I find myself smiling. It's a new chapter, I realize. And for the first time in a long time, I'm excited to see how the story unfolds.

A Gift Beyond Measure: The Day of Revelation

The morning light filters through the blinds of my home office, casting long shadows across my desk. I've been up since dawn, my mind too full of the day ahead to allow for sleep. My hands tremble slightly as I set up my phone to record, a mixture of excitement and nervous energy coursing through my veins.

This video, I know, will be different from all the others I've made during this long journey. Today, I finally get to share the news I've been holding close to my heart for months. Today, I get to reveal the identity of the person who's giving me a second chance at life.

I take a deep breath, centering myself before I begin. The weight of this moment, the culmination of six months of hope and fear, tests and procedures, waiting and praying, settles over me like a warm blanket.

"All right, good morning," I begin, my voice steadier than I feel. "I'm posting this update this morning because I've got some great news and today is a really great day that's been at least 6 months in the making."

As I speak, my mind drifts back to those dark days in November 2023. The sterile smell of the hospital room, the constant beeping of monitors, the gnawing fear that had become my constant companion - it all comes rushing back with vivid clarity.

"When I first became really sick back in November of 2023, I went to the hospital for about eight days," I continue, the memories playing like a movie in my head. "And in the middle of that time, a friend among many friends came to visit me. They immediately offered to donate a kidney for me. I was overwhelmed with gratitude."

I pause, remembering the shock of that moment. The way the world seemed to tilt on its axis, how hope bloomed in my chest for the first time in what felt like forever.

"But they had a real desire to help because they had a family member that had done the same thing before," I explain, marveling at the ripple effect of kindness. "At the time, they didn't want me to reveal their name, and I fully understood that they wanted privacy."

I think about the months that followed, the roller coaster of emotions as we navigated the complex world of organ donation. "But they've gone through all the steps," I say, my voice filled with awe. "They've gone through testing; they've gone through multiple sessions of blood work and procedures."

As I detail the process we're going through, I'm struck anew by the intricacies of modern medicine and the selflessness of my donor. "The process that we're going through is one in which my donor can donate in advance, giving me sort of a credit, a kidney credit, even though we're not a match. But ironically, we are a blood type match, but we're not a tissue match."

My heart races as I approach the crux of my announcement. The moment I've been waiting for, preparing for, for so long. "What that means today, and it's happening right now, my donor is undergoing surgery and is really giving me a second chance at life," I say, my voice thick with emotion. "And at the time she didn't want to share her name but she is ready now."

I take a deep breath, savoring this moment. The reveal of a hero, of a friend who's gone above and beyond anything I could have imagined. "It's my friend Maggie Meador," I finally say, a smile breaking across my face. "She is a big member of the Austin theater community and I can't say enough about how grateful I am for her and for everything she's doing for me."

As I speak Maggie's name, I'm transported back to that day in November when she first made her offer. The memory washes over me, as vivid as if it were happening now...

The hospital room is dim, the afternoon sun barely penetrating the drawn curtains. The air is heavy with the scent of disinfectant, a constant reminder of where I am and why. I'm propped up in bed, feeling weak and scared, but determined to document this journey. The familiar weight of my phone in my hand is comforting as I hit record.

"Hey," I say to the camera, my voice raspier than usual. "One thing that makes my stay here better while I'm fighting for my kidneys, and fighting for my health is the great personal friends that are coming here to visit."

I pan the camera to my left, where Maggie stands, her presence a bright spot in the sterile hospital room. Her smile is warm, her eyes twinkling with a mix of concern and affection that makes my heart swell.

"And I have one of my great friends, Maggie Meador," I continue. "Maggie, tell us why you're here."

Maggie's smile widens, a beacon of normalcy in this clinical setting. "I am here to see my good friend Marc and say hi," she says simply.

"Hello," I respond, touched by her understated kindness. But there's something in her eyes, a determination that tells me there's more to come.

And I'm right. Maggie's expression becomes more serious, more resolute. "And stop it, Marc," she says, her voice firm but gentle. "We all need you back in Austin, just as soon as possible and back with us. But I'm just here to give him the gift of a possible kidney."

Her words hit me like a physical force. I feel my breath catch, my eyes widening in disbelief. The world seems to stop spinning for a moment as the magnitude of what she's offering sinks in.

"That has blown my mind," I manage to say, my voice thick with emotion. "We're still in the early stages but you know that you guys are among the best people that I've ever met and known. Thank you for coming and sharing that gift with me."

As I end the recording, I'm overwhelmed by the magnitude of what Maggie has just offered. In this moment of darkness, she's offered a beacon of hope, a lifeline I never expected. It's more than just a kidney - it's a chance at life, at a future I was beginning to think I might not have.

Back in the present, I blink away the tears that have formed as I relived that powerful memory. The emotion of that day, the hope that Maggie's offer ignited, is just as strong now as it was then.

"But she should be in surgery right now," I continue, my voice wavering slightly. The reality of what's happening at this very moment - Maggie undergoing major surgery for me - is almost too much to comprehend. "And I'll stop by the hospital later on to visit her."

As I wrap up the recording, mentioning the food drive to help with Maggie's recovery, I'm struck by the journey we've been on since that day in the hospital. From a moment of despair to this day of hope and new beginnings. It's been a road filled with challenges, setbacks, and moments of doubt. But through it all, Maggie's offer has been a constant source of hope, a light guiding me through the darkest times.

"Once again Maggie, I can't thank you enough for the gift that you're giving me, and I'm grateful. Thank you," I conclude, my voice filled with emotion that words can't fully express.

I end the recording and sit back in my chair, letting out a long breath. The magnitude of this moment, of Maggie's gift, settles over me like a warm blanket. It's more than just a kidney. It's hope, it's life, it's a second chance I never dared to dream of.

As I prepare to head to the hospital to see Maggie, I'm filled with a sense of purpose and gratitude that goes beyond anything I've ever experienced. This is a new chapter, not just in my health journey, but in my understanding of human kindness and connection.

I think about the long road ahead - the surgery, the recovery, the lifelong commitment to anti-rejection medications. But for the first time in a long time, I'm not afraid. Whatever challenges lie ahead, I know I'll face them with renewed strength, buoyed by the incredible gift Maggie has given me.

The journey isn't over. In many ways, it's just beginning. But thanks to Maggie, thanks to the power of friendship and selflessness, the road ahead looks brighter than I ever imagined possible. As I grab my keys and head for the door, I'm filled with a sense of hope and possibility that I haven't felt in years.

Today, Maggie is giving me a kidney. But what she's really giving me is so much more - a future, a second chance, a new lease on life. And I'm determined to make the most of it, to honor her gift in every way I can.

As I step out into the sunlight, I take a deep breath, savoring the moment. Today is the first day of my new life. And I'm ready for whatever comes next.

Chapter 25: The Long Wait: June's Bitter Truth

The early June sun streams through my office window, casting a warm glow on my desk. It's been almost a month since Maggie's surgery, a month of anticipation and hope. My fingers tremble slightly as I dial the number for the Abdominal Transplant Clinic, my heart racing with excitement. Surely, I think, today will be the day I get news about my exchange kidney.

The phone rings twice before a familiar voice answers. "Abdominal Transplant Clinic, this is Sarah. How can I help you?"

"Hi Sarah, it's Marc Majcher," I say, trying to keep my voice steady. "I'm calling to check on the status of my exchange kidney. As you know, my friend Maggie donated on my behalf last month, and I was wondering if there's been any progress on finding a match for me."

There's a pause on the other end of the line, and I feel my stomach clench. "Marc," Sarah begins, her voice gentle but professional, "I'm glad you called. I know you're eager for news, but I want to set realistic expectations for you."

I lean back in my chair, a sense of unease creeping over me. "What do you mean?" I ask, my earlier excitement giving way to apprehension.

Sarah takes a breath before continuing. "The exchange process can take some time, Marc. While Maggie's donation has significantly improved your position, it usually takes anywhere from three months to a year to fulfill the original recipient's kidney match, depending on several factors."

Her words hit me like a physical blow. Three months to a year? The room seems to spin for a moment as I process this information. "I... I didn't realize," I stammer, struggling to keep my composure. "I thought... I guess I thought it would be sooner."

"I understand," Sarah says, her voice sympathetic. "It's a complex process, and every case is unique. We're doing everything we can to find your perfect match as quickly as possible."

We talk for a few more minutes, Sarah explaining more about the exchange process and reassuring me that they haven't forgotten about me. But her words wash over me in a blur, my mind still reeling from the realization that my wait is far from over.

As I hang up the phone, I feel a wave of emotions threatening to overwhelm me. Disappointment, frustration, fear - they all swirl together, creating a knot in my chest that makes it hard to breathe. I stand up abruptly, needing to move, to do something to dispel this restless energy.

I pace the length of my office, my mind racing. How do I face this news? How do I tell my family, my friends, who have been so supportive, so hopeful? And Maggie - oh God,

Maggie. The thought of her sacrifice, of the pain she went through, now seems to weigh on me even more heavily.

I stop at the window, looking out at the sunny day that now seems to mock my dark mood. "Get it together, Marc," I mutter to myself, pressing my forehead against the cool glass. "This is just another hurdle. You've faced worse."

But even as I try to rally my spirits, I can feel a heaviness settling over me. The road ahead, which had seemed so bright and full of promise just moments ago, now stretches out long and uncertain before me.

I take a deep breath, squaring my shoulders. I can't let this setback defeat me. I owe it to Maggie, to my family, to myself, to stay strong, to keep fighting. But as I turn away from the window, I can't shake the feeling that I'm settling in for a long, difficult wait.

The dialysis machine in the corner of the room, ever-present and unyielding, seems to mock me with its steady hum. It's a reminder of the reality I'm still facing, the daily struggle that isn't over yet. Not by a long shot.

I sit back down at my desk, my eyes falling on the calendar. June stretches out before me, followed by July, August, September... How many of these months will pass before I get the call I'm waiting for? How many more days of dialysis, of fatigue, of putting my life on hold?

But I can't think like that. I won't. I reach for my phone again, this time to call Teri. I need to share this news, to lean on her strength. As the phone rings, I steel myself. This is just another chapter in this long journey. And I'm determined to see it through, no matter how long it takes.

The wait continues, but so does my fight. One day at a time, one hurdle at a time. That's how I'll get through this. That's how I'll make it to the other side.

Chapter 26: Summer of Uncertainty

The Texas summer arrives with its usual ferocity, the heat settling over Austin like a heavy blanket. As the temperatures soar outside, I find myself in a strange limbo, my days a blur of dialysis, exercise, and an ever-present undercurrent of waiting.

Early mornings become my sanctuary. I rise before the sun, strapping on my helmet and wheeling my mountain bike out of the garage. The streets are quiet, the air still cool from the night. As I pedal, I can almost pretend that everything is normal, that I'm just another guy out for a morning ride.

But reality always creeps in. My breath comes faster than it should, my muscles protesting more quickly than they once did. Still, I push on, each rotation of the pedals a small act of defiance against my failing body.

"You're looking good out there," a neighbor calls one morning as I pass. I raise a hand in greeting, mustering a smile. If only they knew, I think. If only they could see the exhaustion that settles into my bones after each ride, the way I have to rest for hours afterward just to function.

The dialysis center becomes a second home, its sterile walls and humming machines a constant in my life. I chat with the nurses, exchange nods with the other patients. We're all in this waiting game together, though few of them know the added weight I carry.

"Any news?" one of the regulars asks me one day, his eyes kind behind his thick glasses.

I shake my head, forcing a smile. "Not yet," I say, the words tasting bitter on my tongue. "But soon, hopefully."

As July bleeds into August, I find myself grappling with a growing fear. What if I'm unmatchable? The thought creeps in during quiet moments, a sinister whisper in the back of my mind. My blood type, O+, once a point of pride as a universal donor, now feels like a curse. I can only receive from other O+ donors, a fact that narrows my options significantly.

And then there are the transfusions. Seven of them between October and November of last year, each one increasing the antibodies in my blood. I remember the doctors explaining it to me, their voices grave. "It makes finding a match more difficult," they'd said. "And even receiving blood in an emergency becomes more complicated."

The weight of this knowledge sits heavy on my chest, a constant companion to the physical discomfort of my failing kidneys.

It's my dialysis social worker who suggests therapy. "It might help to talk to someone," she says gently one day, sliding a card across the table to me. "Someone outside of all this."

I stare at the card for a long moment before pocketing it. I've never been one for therapy, always priding myself on my ability to handle things on my own. But as the days wear on, as the waiting stretches endlessly before me, I find myself dialing the number.

Dr. Simmons' office is cozy, all warm colors and soft furnishings. It's a stark contrast to the clinical settings I've become so accustomed to. As I settle into the plush armchair across from her, I find the words spilling out of me, a torrent of fear and frustration and guilt that I've kept bottled up for so long.

"I feel like I'm letting everyone down," I admit in one session, my voice barely above a whisper. "Maggie gave me this incredible gift, and I'm still... still stuck."

Dr. Simmons leans forward, her eyes kind. "You're not letting anyone down, Marc," she says firmly. "This waiting period is part of the process. It's okay to struggle with it."

Her words are a balm to my battered spirit, but the guilt lingers. It's there in the pit of my stomach when well-meaning friends congratulate me on my "new kidney," not understanding that the exchange is still pending.

"Oh, actually," I find myself saying again and again, "I'm still waiting. The exchange process can take some time."

I see the confusion in their eyes, the slight falter in their smiles. I hasten to explain, to reassure them that yes, Maggie's donation was successful, and yes, it's greatly improved my chances. But with each explanation, I feel a little piece of myself wearing away.

The physical pain is a constant companion, ebbing and flowing but never truly absent. There are days when it's all I can do to get out of bed, to go through the motions of living. But I push through, hiding the worst of it from my family, from Teri. They worry enough, I tell myself. They don't need to see this darkness.

As August draws to a close and September looms on the horizon, I find myself standing in front of the bathroom mirror late one night. The face that looks back at me is drawn, tired in a way that goes beyond physical exhaustion.

"You can do this," I whisper to my reflection, the words a mantra I've repeated countless times over the summer. "You're strong enough. You can wait."

But as I turn away from the mirror, I can't shake the feeling that I'm lying to myself. The wait stretches before me, endless and uncertain. And for the first time since this all began, I allow myself to wonder: what if my kidney never comes?

The thought sends a shiver through me, a cold fear that settles in my bones. I push it away, forcing myself to focus on the present. One day at a time, I remind myself. That's all I can do.

As I settle into bed, Teri's steady breathing beside me a comforting rhythm, I close my eyes and try to picture the future. A future where I'm healthy, where the wait is over. It's harder to see than it once was, the image blurry and indistinct.

But it's there. And as I drift off to sleep, I cling to that faint image, that distant hope. It's all I have to hold onto in this summer of uncertainty.

Chapter 27: The Call That Changed Everything

October arrives with a whisper, the Texas heat finally beginning to loosen its grip. The changing season brings with it a sense of melancholy that I can't quite shake. It's been nearly five months since Maggie's donation, five months of waiting, hoping, and trying not to lose faith.

I've settled into a routine, one that feels both comforting and suffocating. Dialysis three times a week, therapy sessions, morning bike rides when I have the energy. The days blend together, a monotonous cycle of medical appointments and quiet desperation.

On the morning of October 7th, I wake early, the pre-dawn darkness still clinging to the world outside. I lie in bed for a moment, listening to Teri's soft breathing beside me, steeling myself for another day of waiting.

My mountain bike calls to me, but my body protests. The fatigue that's become my constant companion weighs heavily on me this morning. Instead, I make my way to my home office, figuring I might as well get some work done.

The clock on my computer reads 11:58 AM when my phone rings. The caller ID flashes "Abdominal Transplant Clinic," and my heart leaps into my throat. I've received so many calls from them over the months, each one a rollercoaster of hope and disappointment. I take a deep breath, trying to temper my expectations as I answer.

"Hello, this is Marc," I say, proud of how steady my voice sounds.

"Hello Marc, this is Sarah from the Abdominal Transplant Clinic. I have some important news for you."

There's something in her tone, a hint of excitement that makes my pulse quicken. I grip the edge of my desk, my knuckles turning white.

"Yes, go ahead," I manage to say, my voice barely above a whisper.

"We've found a living donor match for you, Marc. We'd like to schedule your transplant surgery for October 24th at 5 AM."

The world seems to stop spinning for a moment. I can hear Sarah's voice, but her words don't make sense. A match? Surgery? It can't be real.

"Are... are you serious?" I stammer, my voice trembling.

"Yes, Marc. This is real," Sarah confirms, and I can hear the smile in her voice. "We also need you to come in for a pre-op visit on October 17th. Can you make those dates work?"

Tears well up in my eyes, blurring my vision. "Yes, absolutely. I'll be there," I say, choking back a sob. "Thank you... thank you so much."

"You're welcome, Marc. We'll send you all the details via email. Congratulations."

As I hang up the phone, a wave of emotion crashes over me. Joy, relief, disbelief, gratitude - they all swirl together, overwhelming in their intensity. I sit in stunned silence for a moment, my mind struggling to process what just happened.

Then, suddenly, I can't sit still any longer. I stand up abruptly, my chair clattering to the floor behind me. I need to move, to breathe, to shout this news from the rooftops.

I race down the stairs, taking them two at a time, my feet barely touching the ground. I burst through the front door, the cool October air hitting my face like a splash of water, grounding me in this moment.

Standing on the sidewalk, I look up at the clear blue sky, tears streaming down my face. I spread my arms wide, as if trying to embrace the entire world.

"Thank you!" I shout, my voice ringing out in the quiet neighborhood. "Thank you for everything!"

I spin around, laughing and crying at the same time. The emotions I've kept bottled up for so long come pouring out in a cathartic release.

"All the hurdles, all the pain..." I say to myself, my voice choked with emotion. "It was worth it. Maggie, my family, my friends... I couldn't have done this without you."

I notice a neighbor walking their dog, staring at me with a mixture of concern and curiosity. Under normal circumstances, I might feel embarrassed by my public display of emotion. But not today. Today, I want to share my joy with the world.

"Everything okay, Marc?" the neighbor calls out.

I beam at them, my face wet with tears but split by the widest grin I've worn in months. "Everything's perfect," I reply. "I'm getting a new kidney. I'm getting a second chance at life."

The neighbor smiles and gives me a thumbs up, and I'm struck by how such a simple gesture can mean so much in this moment.

I take a deep breath, trying to compose myself, but I can't wipe the smile off my face. My mind is already racing ahead, thinking of all the people I need to tell, all the preparations I need to make.

"October 24th," I whisper to myself. "A new beginning."

As I turn to walk back into the house, ready to share the news with Teri and start preparing for the life-changing surgery ahead, I'm filled with a sense of hope and excitement I haven't felt in years.

The wait isn't over yet - there are still 17 days until the surgery. But for the first time in a long time, I can see the finish line. The journey has been long and difficult, filled with more setbacks and challenges than I ever could have imagined. But standing here, on the precipice of a new chapter in my life, I know that every moment of struggle has led me to this point.

I take one last look at the sky, feeling a profound sense of gratitude wash over me. For Maggie's selfless gift, for the doctors and nurses who've cared for me, for my family and friends who've supported me every step of the way. For the stranger who's about to give me a second chance at life.

As I step back into the house, I'm ready to face whatever comes next. The pre-op appointment, the surgery itself, the long recovery ahead - I'll tackle it all with renewed strength and determination. Because now, finally, the wait is almost over. And a new life is waiting just around the corner.

Chapter 28: A Perspective on Waiting

As the days count down to my pre-op appointment, I find myself reflecting not just on the past year, but on my entire journey with kidney failure. The pain and frustration of this year-long wait have been immense, but I'm acutely aware that my experience is far from the norm. Many patients spend multiple years, even decades, waiting for a match. Some never make it onto the list at all.

This realization brings me back to my first bout with kidney failure, a harrowing three-year ordeal from 2009 to 2012 that nearly cost me my life several times. The contrast between then and now is stark, a testament to how much has changed in the healthcare landscape - and how much still needs to change.

One quiet evening, as I'm setting up my nightly dialysis, the memories of those early days come flooding back. I remember the fear, the confusion, the feeling of being utterly lost in a system that seemed designed to let me fall through the cracks.

In May 2009, when my kidneys first failed, there was no Affordable Care Act. I was uninsured, scared, and rapidly deteriorating. Those first six months, from May until my birthday on November 2nd, nearly killed me. I can still feel the swelling, the breathlessness, the creeping certainty that I was dying.

I think about the doctor in Austin who took my cash payments and prescribed me prednisone - a massive dose for my then 300-pound, fluid-filled body. I remember how quickly the fluid dropped off, leaving me at 208 pounds in a matter of days. But the prednisone dose never changed, leading to steroid psychosis - a horrifying experience I wouldn't wish on anyone.

When that doctor left for Italy, leaving me without care, I turned to public clinics. Their response? Six-month follow-ups. They might as well have handed me a death sentence. I became a frequent flyer at the emergency room, desperate for help. I can still hear the voice of one doctor, his words etched in my memory: "We're not checking you in or keeping you because you're not insured." At the time, I thought he was being cruel. Now, I realize he was just being honest about a cruel system.

It was my mother who saved me, insisting I leave Austin and move to the Rio Grande Valley. There, she introduced me to a Nigerian nephrologist who saw me not just as a patient, but as a person - a younger brother in need of help. This doctor fought for me every step of the way - to get me on dialysis, to secure funding and insurance, to get me on the transplant list. He advocated for me during every crisis, literally saving my life four times. Without him, I'm certain I wouldn't have made it to Christmas 2009.

The contrast between then and now is striking. Today, I have insurance. I have a team of doctors who know my name, who treat me like a person rather than a problem. I have access to regular care, to necessary medications, to the hope of a transplant. The Affordable Care Act, for all its imperfections, has made a world of difference.

Yet even as I appreciate how far I've come, I'm acutely aware of how far we still have to go. How many others are out there now, facing what I faced in 2009? How many are being told to wait six months for a follow-up when they might not survive six weeks? How many are being turned away from emergency rooms, their pain and fear dismissed because they lack insurance?

This perspective makes the pain and frustration of the past year feel different. Yes, it's been hard. Yes, there have been moments of despair, of feeling like the wait would never end. But I've had care. I've had support. I've had hope.

As I finish setting up my dialysis for the night, I find myself filled with a complex mix of emotions. Gratitude for how far I've come. Hope for the surgery that lies ahead. But also a deep, abiding concern for those still caught in the cracks of our healthcare system.

I close my eyes, listening to the familiar hum of the dialysis machine. "Thank you," I whisper, my words meant for my mother, for that Nigerian doctor who saw me as a person, for everyone who's helped me reach this point. "And I'm sorry," I add, thinking of all those still waiting, still struggling, still invisible to a system that should be designed to help them.

As I drift off to sleep, I make a silent promise to myself. When this is over, when I'm healthy again, I'll find a way to help. To advocate for change. To be for others what that Nigerian doctor was for me - a voice, a fighter, a lifeline.

The wait isn't just about me anymore. It's about all of us. And somehow, that makes it easier to bear.

CHAPTER 29- The Night Before: A Mother's Wisdom

The hotel lounge is softly lit, creating an intimate atmosphere that feels separate from the world outside. Tomorrow morning, I'll be in surgery, but right now, sitting here with my mother, Mary George, time seems to slow down. Teri films quietly from across the table, capturing this moment for posterity.

I study my mother's face, noting the familiar determination in her eyes. After decades in healthcare as a pharmacist, she carries herself with the measured confidence of someone who has seen both the best and worst of our medical system.

"So I'm here with my mom, Mary George," I begin, trying to keep my voice light. "She's been traveling around the state because she has grandkids in Austin, grandkids in Houston..."

But there are deeper questions weighing on my mind, questions that feel urgent on this eve of transformation. I lean forward, my tone growing more serious.

"Just to get back on the health issue... what do you think the challenges would be like if either Dominic or myself didn't have resources like insurance?"

My mother's response is immediate and stark. "You guys would be dead."

The bluntness of her answer catches me off guard, though I know it's true. She leans forward, her eyes intense with the weight of past memories.

"Because what I think... even without insurance, before you had insurance, well, it's a good thing you met Dr. Sanusi who was more interested in taking care of you, treating you, than making money off of you. If it was a doctor interested in making money, he would have written you off."

She pauses, reflecting on those difficult days. "Two, I had a job that gave me flexibility. Because I lived close to the hospital, sometimes I could spend the night there with you, then go home, take my shower, go to work."

"Do you think that's true for the average American family?" I ask, although I already know the answer.

My mother shakes her head, her expression grave. "I was fortunate. As a pharmacist, I was working at a clinic where people understood what health issues can bring. They know it's not something to take lightly."

As she describes her clinic - the comprehensive care they provided, the diverse patient population they served - I can hear the passion in her voice growing stronger. Her years of experience have given her a front-row seat to the healthcare crisis in America.

"Many patients didn't have insurance through their work," she continues. "Some worked as laborers, as caregivers - jobs that don't provide insurance. If they went to a private physician, they wouldn't be taken care of. But the clinic took very good care of them."

I seize this moment to ask the question that's been on my mind, especially given my own journey. "What would you say to somebody who feels it's not government's responsibility to contribute to programs like your clinic or maintain something like the Affordable Care Act?"

My mother's response is firm and immediate. "I think it's the government's responsibility. Not only for clinics but for public health. Every country I know provides these two basic things: education and healthcare. It shouldn't be connected to your job."

She leans back, drawing on her extensive international experience. "I've been to many countries - Canada, countries in Europe. They all have public health. Your work has nothing to do with your health insurance."

Her voice takes on a more personal tone as she continues. "I've been in situations myself where as soon as I quit a job, my insurance vanished. If I were to have a heart attack between jobs, that would be it. That shouldn't be. This is an issue that affects everybody, from a two-month-old baby to a 90-year-old."

I glance at my watch, aware of the early morning that awaits me. "Mom, I'm not going to talk to you much longer since I have to be up there at 3:00 tomorrow..."

But she has one more thing to say, reaching for my hand as she speaks. "Healthcare is so expensive. People should be able to get healthcare regardless of their financial status. If you want something else, you get something else, but it should be available. It should be there."

I nod, emotion welling up in my throat. My mother's words carry the weight of both personal experience and professional wisdom. Tomorrow, I'll receive a kidney transplant - a possibility that exists only because of insurance, because of dedicated healthcare providers, because of a system that, while flawed, at least gave me a chance.

As we sit there in the soft light of the hotel lounge, the reality of tomorrow's surgery hangs in the air between us. But so does something else - the understanding that my story, our story, is part of a larger narrative about healthcare in America. About who gets care and who doesn't. About who lives and who dies.

My mother squeezes my hand one more time, and in that gesture, I feel decades of love, worry, and determination. Tomorrow will bring its own challenges, but tonight, I'm grateful for this moment of clarity and connection. For a mother's wisdom that extends beyond personal care to encompass a vision of what healthcare could and should be for everyone.

CHAPTER 30: The Final Countdown

The world feels different at 2:30 AM, as if suspended between reality and dreams. Streetlights cast intermittent shadows across the dashboard as Teri drives us toward the hospital. The familiar roads look alien in the pre-dawn darkness, as if we're traveling not just through space but through time itself - leaving behind the person I was and moving toward whoever I'll become after today's surgery.

"Remember Teri," I say to the camera, my voice soft in the quiet car, "my lovely wife who's been with me this whole journey and before... I think it's wonderful that we're basically about a year past the initial nightmare of November 8th, 2023."

The symmetry of the timing strikes me - how life has a way of coming full circle. I turn to Teri, emotion thick in my throat. "What, if anything, has this taught you?"

Her eyes stay fixed on the road, but I can see them glistening in the dashboard lights. "Um, how strong we are," she says, her voice wavering slightly. "That we can get through anything. I mean, I've always been a caretaker but... kind of just learning more of a personal caretaker role."

She pauses, collecting herself. "This match came as a total surprise. The timing... yes. I was at work and I didn't even look at my phone until I got in the car for lunch. I just started crying."

My heart swells with love and gratitude. "I just want to say I love you so much and I can't imagine making it through this without you. Thank you so much. I love you."

I look down at the small stress ball Teri gave me - a mini punching bag to help with last-minute anxiety. But what I'm feeling goes beyond anxiety. It's something deeper, more primal.

"I have to be honest..." I begin, trying to put words to the strange sensations coursing through my body. "I don't know if it's psychosis or what, but I'm feeling like everything's winding down, you know? My voice is a little bit croaky. I just feel aches in my bones and my shoulders."

I pause, searching for the right words. "I know that won't go away immediately with the surgery, but I just feel like my body is preparing itself for new help and saying a final salute to the parts that did their best but couldn't make it through this journey."

As we drive on through the darkness, I'm acutely aware of every sensation, every breath, every beat of my failing kidneys. In a few hours, everything will change. The thought is both terrifying and exhilarating.

The hospital waiting room at 5:10 AM feels like a liminal space, existing somewhere between night and day, between the old life and the new. Teri sits alone, speaking to her phone camera after they've taken me back for surgery.

"They just took him back to surgery, so it's officially about to start," she says, her voice a mixture of excitement and nervousness. "It's very exciting... nervous." She takes a deep breath, steadying herself. "It should last probably like 4 hours. It's a pretty long procedure. Obviously, it's pretty big. About 15, 10-15 maybe 20% anxious and the rest just very excited. This is going to change our lives."

A smile crosses her face as she remembers our final exchange. "On our way here I asked Marc what and how he was feeling, and his response was... 'I'm determined.' I thought that was a great answer."

Time moves strangely in hospital waiting rooms. Minutes stretch into hours, then suddenly collapse into moments. At 9:00 AM, Teri's face appears on camera again, this time transformed by joy.

"I have an update!" she exclaims, emotion making her voice tremble. "I got off the phone with the surgeon just a minute ago and Marc is done with the surgery. She said he did amazing - the kidney is working perfectly!"

Her expression becomes more serious as she continues, "The next 24 hours is vital, and what we need to watch closest, make sure everything keeps working correctly. But she's going to come up here in like 20 or 30 minutes to actually talk to me in person. But he's done! Oh my gosh... feels good."

The late afternoon sun filters through the hospital room window, casting a gentle glow over everything. I lie in the bed, tired but content, feeling both completely different and exactly the same. The pain is there, yes, but there's something else too - a sense of renewal, of possibility.

I pick up my phone one last time, knowing this will be the final scene of this chapter of my life. "Hey everybody, it's Marc," I say softly, my voice rough but steady. "I'm about six or seven hours out of surgery. I'm doing pretty well - the surgery was a complete success."

I shift slightly, wincing at the pain. "I'm just dealing with some pain now and some blood pressure issues, but they're getting that all into control."

Emotion wells up in my throat as I think about everything and everyone that has brought me to this moment. "I thank you guys all for your well wishes and for your great support over the last year. I might do without a lot of visitors the next few days, if that's okay, just because the pain and the recovery is still a little bit... bit of a challenge."

A weak smile crosses my face. "I don't know if that was proper grammar or not, but it don't matter at this point. I'm living with a new kidney and hopefully another few decades."

Looking directly into the camera, I feel the weight of this moment, the end of one journey and the beginning of another. "Thank you guys. Bye."

As I set the phone down, I'm aware that this is more than just the end of a documentary. It's the end of a chapter in my life - a chapter filled with pain and fear, yes, but also with love, support, and incredible acts of kindness. And now, thanks to modern medicine, skilled surgeons, and the generosity of others, I'm beginning a new chapter.

The sun continues its slow descent outside my window, casting long shadows across my hospital room. I close my eyes, feeling the various aches and pains, but also feeling something new - hope, pure and simple. Whatever comes next, I know I'm ready for it. This is my eighth day, my new beginning. And I'm determined to make the most of it.

www.ingramcontent.com/pod-product-compliance
Lightning Source LLC
Chambersburg PA
CBHW031623210526
45464CB00004B/1718